Lecture Notes in Bioinformatics 3886

Edited by S. Istrail, P. Pevzner, and M. Waterman

Editorial Board: A. Apostolico   S. Brunak   M. Gelfand
T. Lengauer   S. Miyano   G. Myers   M.-F. Sagot   D. Sankoff
R. Shamir   T. Speed   M. Vingron   W. Wong

Subseries of Lecture Notes in Computer Science

Eric G. Bremer   Jörg Hakenberg
Eui-Hong (Sam) Han   Daniel Berrar
Werner Dubitzky (Eds.)

Knowledge Discovery in Life Science Literature

PAKDD 2006 International Workshop, KDLL 2006
Singapore, April 9, 2006
Proceedings

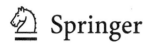 Springer

Series Editors

Sorin Istrail, Brown University, Providence, RI, USA
Pavel Pevzner, University of California, San Diego, CA, USA
Michael Waterman, University of Southern California, Los Angeles, CA, USA

Volume Editors

Eric G. Bremer
Children's Memorial Hospital, Brain Tumor Research Program
2300 Children's Plaza, Chicago, Illinois 60614, USA
E-mail: egbremer@northwestern.edu

Jörg Hakenberg
Humbold-Universität zu Berlin
Computer Science Department, Knowledge Management in Bioinformatics
Unter den Linden 6, 10099 Berlin, Germany
E-mail: hakenberg@informatik.hu-berlin.de

Eui-Hong (Sam) Han
iXmatch Inc.
5555 West 78th Street Suite E, Minneapolis, MN 55439-2702, USA
E-mail: han@cs.umn.edu

Daniel Berrar
Werner Dubitzky
University of Ulster
School of Biomedial Sciences, Bioinformatics Research Group
Cromore Road, Coleraine BT52 1SA, Northern Ireland, UK
E-mail: {dp.berrar,w.dubitzky}@ulster.ac.uk

Library of Congress Control Number: 2006921543

CR Subject Classification (1998): H.2.8, J.3, I.2, H.3, I.5, I.4, F.1

LNCS Sublibrary: SL 8 – Bioinformatics

ISSN	0302-9743
ISBN-10	3-540-32809-2 Springer Berlin Heidelberg New York
ISBN-13	978-3-540-32809-4 Springer Berlin Heidelberg New York

Springer is a part of Springer Science+Business Media

springer.com

© Springer-Verlag Berlin Heidelberg 2006
Printed in Germany

Typesetting: Camera-ready by author, data conversion by Scientific Publishing Services, Chennai, India
Printed on acid-free paper   SPIN: 11683568   06/3142   5 4 3 2 1 0

Preface

This volume of the Springer Lecture Notes in Computer Science series contains the contributions presented at the International Workshop on Knowledge Discovery Life Science Literature 2006 (KDLL 2006) held in Singapore, 9 April 2006, in conjunction with the 10th Pacific-Asia Conference on Knowledge Discovery and Data Mining (PAKDD 2006).

The life sciences encompass research and development in areas such as biology, pharmacology, biophysics, biochemistry, neuroscience, medicine, and environmental sciences. A common theme among life science disciplines is the desire to understand the stimuli-response mechanisms of biological entities, systems, and processes at different levels of organization—from molecules to organisms to ecosystems. As natural phenomena are being probed and mapped in ever-greater detail, life scientists are generating an increasingly growing amount of textual information in the form of full-text research articles, abstracts, Web content, reports, books, and so on. Even in well-focused subject areas it is becoming more and more difficult for researchers and practitioners to find, read, and process all textual information relevant to their tasks. Knowledge discovery in text (KDT) is a fast-developing field that encompasses a variety of methodologies, methods and tools, which facilitate automated processing of text information stored in electronic format. KDT tasks that are particularly interesting to life science include:

- Identification and retrieval of relevant documents from one or more large collections of documents;
- Identification of relevant sections in large documents (passage retrieval);
- Co-reference resolution, i.e., the identification of expressions in texts that refer to the same biological, medical, or biotechnological entity, process, or activity;
- Extraction of life science entities (e.g., genes, proteins, agonists, antagonists, mechanisms, disease, etc.) or relationships (e.g., gene-function, drug–gene interactions, protein–protein interactions, diseases and disease states, etc.) from text collections;
- Automated characterization of biological, biomedical, and biotechnological entities and processes (e.g., annotation of genes or proteins);
- Extraction and characterization of more complex patterns and interaction networks (e.g., biological pathways, topologies, reaction networks, drug-response patterns);
- Automated generation of text summaries;
- Automated construction, expansion, and curation of ontologies for different domains (e.g., characterization of genes, proteins, medical terms);
- Construction of controlled vocabularies from fixed sets of documents for particular domains in biology and medicine.

KDT approaches in the life sciences are faced with a number of challenges that make such endeavors much more complicated than KDT studies in classical application areas such as retail, marketing, customer relationship management, and finance. Important challenges of KDT approaches in biology, biochemistry, biotechnology, medicine, and other life science areas include:

- The need for a mechanistic understanding of biology at different levels of organization and therefore the need for descriptive, predictive as well as for explanatory models;
- The requirement to handle large terminologies characteristics for life science areas. Such terminologies are often redundant, inconsistent, and are constantly evolving;
- The necessity to process and analyze life science texts at different levels of unit granularity, e.g., abstract, full text, passage, section of text such as results, discussion, conclusion sections;
- The management and handling of KDT data and KDT results – this includes the access to and integration of text collections in particular in heterogeneous and distributed computing environments such as the Internet, intranets and grids;
- The complex issue of pre-processing and transforming life science texts using statistical, natural language processing, and other techniques. This also involves issues such as combination of life science text with other forms of data and information, e.g., data from biomedical experiments and information from ontologies, thesauri, dictionaries, warehouses and similar systems;
- The adaptation and improvement of existing and development of new methodologies, algorithms, tools, and systems for different KDT tasks, such as text clustering, classification, entity and relationship extraction, template-based approaches, etc. relevant to life science R&D problems;
- Both the statistical as well as the epistemological (knowledge-based) validation and interpretation of KDT results;
- The constraints posed by computational resources (memory, storage, processor, network bandwidth) arising from large-scale KDT tasks in the life sciences;
- The standardization of KDT approaches in the life sciences.

The objective of the KDLL 2006 Workshop was to bring together scientists who have researched and applied KDT methodologies and techniques in the context of biology, biotechnology, medicine, and other life science areas. The workshop was conceived as a forum facilitating the discussion of innovative work in progress and of important new KDT directions in the life sciences. In addition to life science areas typically associated with bioinformatics (i.e., molecular and cell biology), a specific intention of the workshop was to discuss KDT developments in biochemistry, pharmacology, medicine, neuroscience, environmental sciences, and so on. By sharing the insights, discussing ongoing work and the results that have been achieved, the workshop participants gleaned a comprehensive view of the state of the art in this area and were able to identify emerging and future research issues.

The workshop was structured into a one-day session consisting of two invited talks and 12 presentations of the papers selected for the workshop. Below we briefly summarize the contributions to KDLL 2006.

The contribution of **Tan et al.** addresses the importan t problem of 'aligning' multiple and partially overlapping ontologies. For this they propose an algorithm capable of taking into account ontology structure. **Mathiak et al.** present an interesting picture search engine for life science literature and show how it can be used to improve literature pre-selection. By looking for papers with images (and their textual annotations) concerning the biomedical experiments, they could considerably improve the precision of the retrieval system. **Torii et al.** explore biomedical named entity tagging and evaluate the performance of headwords and suffixes using names from the Unified Medical Language System and in-corporating the GENIA ontology. Their study sheds new light on how named entity tagging performs under different conditions and assumptions. **Eom et al.** present a tree kernel-based method to mine protein–protein interactions from text. Their results suggest that this method learns protein interaction informa-tion through structure patterns and achieves promising results. **Dimililer et al.** investigate a support vector machine approach to identify and automatically annotate named biomedical entities as an extension of the traditional named entity recognition task to special domains. Specifically, they study the effects of using word formation patterns, lexical, morphological, and surface words for this task. **Huang et al.** explore the problem of discovering potential biomedical relationships from text data. To do so, they follow a study that involves 'tempo-ral topic profiles.' Their approach uses MeSH terms from MEDLINE resources. **Jang et al.** study protein name and protein interaction extraction by using an existing full parser without training or tuning. Their approach is based on a so-phisticated substitution-of-words technique and shows that parsing errors can be reduced and parsing precision increased by this sentence simplification method. **Wu et al.** present a robust named entity recognition system based on support vector machines. Testing their system on biomedical data sets, their results show that their approach outperforms relevant competitor methods and, because of its fast execution time, is suitable for real-time applications. **Wang et al.** look at text classification problems involving examples where a small set of labeled positive examples and a very large set of unlabeled examples exist. They present a weighted voting classifier scheme for tackling this problem. **Takeuchi et al.** investigate the problem of mapping different keywords representing the same en-tity of concept to a canonical form. Such a dictionary with canonical entries may contain many invalid entries. The paper presents methods for detecting invalid entries in such a dictionary. The investigation of **Ning et al.** revolves around automatically filtering and assessing erroneous entries in protein databases. This approach is an important contribution to tackling the problem of handling er-rors in biomedical databases. **Natarajan et al.** present a download agent and pre-processing tool, which facilitates the task of accessing, downloading and pre-processing full-text articles. Once fully developed, this tool will be useful for many applications requiring the handling and processing of large full-text research article collections.

We believe that the KDLL 2006 Workshop has made a valuable contribution towards shaping future work in the field of knowledge discovery in life science literature.

Singapore, April 2006

Eric Bremer
Jörg Hakenberg
Eui-Hong (Sam) Han
Daniel Berrar
Werner Dubitzky

Organization

Acknowledgments

KDLL 2006 was sponsored and organized by SPSS Inc.; The DataMiningGrid Consortium (EC grant IST-2004-004475), Northwestern University, Chicago, IL, USA; Humboldt-Universität zu Berlin, Berlin, Germany; iXmatch Inc., Minneapolis, MN, USA; University of Ulster, Coleraine, Northern Ireland, UK. A special thanks goes to the invited speakers—George Karypis, University of Minnesota, MN, USA and Olivier Jouve, SPSS Inc., Paris, France—who reminded us of the mind-boggling breadth and depth of modern life science informatics and the KDT challenges involved. We are indebted to the PAKDD workshop organizers Ah-Hwee Tan, Nanyang Technological University, Singapore and Huan Liu, Arizona State University, USA for their patience and support with all logistical aspects of the workshop. Finally, we would like to extend our gratitude to the members of the KDLL 2006 International Program Committee.

International Program Committee

Eric Bremer, Brain Tumor Research Program, Children's Memorial Hospital, and Feinberg School of Medicine, Northwestern University, Chicago, IL, USA

Jörg Hakenberg, Computer Science Department, Knowledge Management in Bioinformatics, Humboldt-Universität zu Berlin, Germany

Eui-Hong (Sam) Han, iXmatch Inc., Minneapolis, MN, USA

Daniel Berrar, University of Ulster, School of Biomedical Sciences, Bioinformatics Research Group, Coleraine, Northern Ireland, UK

Werner Dubitzky, University of Ulster, School of Biomedical Sciences, Bioinformatics Research Group, Coleraine, Northern Ireland, UK

Christian Blaschke, bioalma, Madrid, Spain

Kevin Bretonnel Cohen, University of Colorado School of Medicine, Aurora, CO, USA

Nigel Collier, National Institute for Informatics, Tokyo, Japan

Anna Divoli, Faculty of Life Sciences and School of Computer Science, University of Manchester, Manchester, UK

Jürgen Franke, DaimlerChrysler, Ulm, Germany

Lynette Hirschman, Information Technology Center, The MITRE Corporation, Bedford, MA, USA

Olivier Jouve, SPSS Inc., Paris, France

Min-Yen Kan, National University of Singapore, Singapore

Harald Kirsch, European Bioinformatics Institute, Hinxton, UK

Irena Koprinska, University of Sydney, School of Information Technologies, Sydney, Australia

Patrick Lambrix, Linköpings Universitet, Sweden

Simon Lin, Robert H. Lurie Comprehensive Cancer Center, Northwestern University, Chicago, IL, USA

Michael N Liebman, Windber Research Institute, Windber, PA, USA

Eric Martin, SPSS Inc., Paris, France

Adeline Nazarenko, LIPN Institut Galilée, University of Paris-Nord, Paris, France

See-Kiong Ng, Institute for Infocomm Research, Singapore

Gerhard Paaß, Fraunhofer Institute for Autonous Intelligence Systems, St. Augustin, Germany

Patrick Ruch, University Hospital of Geneve, Switzerland; National Library of Medicine, Bethesda, USA

Alexander K. Seewald, Austrian Research Institute for Artificial Intelligence, Vienna, Austria

Shusaku Tsumoto, Department of Medical Informatics, Shimane Medical University, School of Medicine, Izumo, Japan

Karin Verspoor, Computational Linguist Knowledge and Information Systems Science Team Computer & Computational Science Division, Los Alamos National Laboratory, Los Alamos, NM, USA

Paul van der Vet, Computer Science Department, University of Twente, Enschede, Netherlands

Sponsors

SPSS, Inc.

The DataMiningGrid Consortium

The University of Minnesota, Minneapolis, MN, USA

iXmatch Inc., Minnesota, Minneapolis, MN, USA

Children's Memorial Hospital, Chicago, IL, USA

Northwestern University, Chicago, IL, USA

Humboldt-Universität zu Berlin, Berlin, Germany

The University of Ulster, Coleraine, Northern Ireland, UK

Table of Contents

Alignment of Biomedical Ontologies Using Life Science Literature

He Tan, Vaida Jakonienė, Patrick Lambrix,
Johan Aberg, and Nahid Shahmehri

Department of Computer and Information Science,
Linköpings universitet, SE-581 83 Linköping, Sweden

Abstract. In recent years many biomedical ontologies have been developed and many of these ontologies contain overlapping information. To be able to use multiple ontologies they have to be aligned. In this paper we propose strategies for aligning ontologies based on life science literature. We propose a basic algorithm as well as extensions that take the structure of the ontologies into account. We evaluate the strategies and compare them with strategies implemented in the alignment system SAMBO. We also evaluate the combination of the proposed strategies and the SAMBO strategies.

1 Introduction

Ontologies (e.g. [Lam04, Gom99]) can be seen as defining the basic terms and relations of a domain of interest, as well as the rules for combining these terms and relations. They are considered to be an important technology for the Semantic Web. Ontologies are used for communication between people and organizations by providing a common terminology over a domain. They provide the basis for interoperability between systems. They can be used for making the content in information sources explicit and serve as an index to a repository of information. Further, they can be used as a basis for integration of information sources and as a query model for information sources. They also support clearly separating domain knowledge from application-based knowledge as well as validation of data sources. The benefits of using ontologies include reuse, sharing and portability of knowledge across platforms, and improved maintainability, documentation, maintenance, and reliability. Overall, ontologies lead to a better understanding of a field and to more effective and efficient handling of information in that field. In the field of bioinformatics the work on biomedical ontologies is recognized as essential in some of the grand challenges of genomics research [CGGG03] and there is much international research cooperation for the development of ontologies (e.g. the Gene Ontology (GO) [GO00] and Open Biomedical Ontologies (OBO) [OBO] efforts) and the use of ontologies for the Semantic Web (e.g. the EU Network of Excellence REWERSE [REWERSE], [Lam05]).

Many ontologies have already been developed and many of these ontologies contain overlapping information. Often we would therefore want to be able to

E.G. Bremer et al. (Eds.): KDLL 2006, LNBI 3886, pp. 1–17, 2006.

use multiple ontologies. For instance, companies may want to use community standard ontologies and use them together with company-specific ontologies. Applications may need to use ontologies from different areas or from different views on one area. Ontology builders may want to use already existing ontologies as the basis for the creation of new ontologies by extending the existing ontologies or by combining knowledge from different smaller ontologies. In each of these cases it is important to know the relationships between the terms (concepts and relations) in the different ontologies. These relationships can also be used in information integration [JL05]. It has been realized that ontology alignment, i.e. finding relationships between terms in the different ontologies, is a major issue and some organizations (e.g. the organization for Standards and Ontologies for Functional Genomics (SOFG)) have started to deal with it.

In this paper we present instance-based strategies for aligning biomedical ontologies. We focus on equivalence and is-a relationships. In section 3 we present an algorithm based on naive Bayes classifiers as well as extensions that take the structure of the ontologies into account. The strategies use life science literature and build on the intuition that a similarity measure between concepts can be computed based on the probability that documents about one concept are also about the other concept. Section 4 describes different experiments regarding the quality and performance of the proposed strategies and the combination of these strategies with other existing strategies. We describe related work in section 5 and conclude the paper in section 6. In the next section we provide background information on biomedical ontologies and ontology alignment systems.

2 Background

2.1 Biomedical Ontologies

In recent years many biomedical ontologies have been developed and the field has matured enough to develop standardization efforts. An example of this is the organization of the first SOFG conference in 2002 and the development of the SOFG resource on ontologies. Further, there exist ontologies that have reached the status of de facto standard and are being used extensively for annotation of databases. Also, OBO was started as an umbrella web address for ontologies for use within the genomics and proteomics domains. Many biomedical ontologies are available via OBO and there are many overlapping ontologies in the field.

The ontologies that we use in this paper are GO ontologies, Signal-Ontology (SigO), Medical Subject Headings (MeSH) and the Anatomical Dictionary for the Adult Mouse (MA). The GO Consortium is a joint project which goal is to produce a structured, precisely defined, common and dynamic controlled vocabulary that describes the roles of genes and proteins in all organisms. Currently, there are three independent ontologies publicly available over the Internet: biological process, molecular function and cellular component. The GO ontologies are a de facto standard and many different bio-data sources are today annotated with GO terms. The terms in GO are arranged as nodes in a directed acyclic graph, where multiple inheritance is allowed. The purpose of the SigO project is to extract common features of cell signaling in the model organisms, try to understand what cell signaling is and how cell signaling systems can be modeled. SigO is a publicly available controlled vocabulary of the cell signaling system. It is based on the knowledge of the Cell Signaling Networks data source [TNK98] and treats complex knowledge of living cells such as pathways, networks and causal relationships among molecules. The ontology consists of a flow diagram of signal transduction and a conceptual hierarchy of biochemical attributes of signaling molecules. MeSH is a controlled vocabulary produced by the American National Library of Medicine and used for indexing, cataloging, and searching for biomedical and health-related information and documents. It consists of sets of terms naming descriptors in a hierarchical structure. These descriptors are organized in 15 categories, such as the category for anatomic terms, which is the category we use in the evaluation. MA is cooperating with the Anatomical Dictionary for Mouse Development to generate an anatomy ontology (controlled vocabulary) covering the lifespan of the laboratory mouse. It organizes anatomical structures spatially and functionally, using is-a and part-of relationships.

2.2   Ontology Alignment Systems

There exist a number of ontology alignment systems that support the user to find inter-ontology relationships. Some of these systems are also ontology merge systems, i.e. they can create a new ontology based on the source ontologies and the alignment relationships. Many ontology alignment systems can be described as instantiations of the general framework defined in [LT05b] (figure 1). An alignment algorithm receives as input two source ontologies. The algorithm can include several matchers. These matchers calculate similarities between the terms from the different source ontologies. The matchers can implement strategies based on linguistic matching, structure-based strategies, constraint-based approaches, instance-based strategies, strategies that use auxiliary information or a combination of these.

Alignment suggestions are then determined by combining and filtering the results generated by one or more matchers. The pairs of terms with a similarity value above a certain threshold are retained as alignment suggestions. By using different matchers and combining them and filtering in different ways we obtain different alignment strategies. The suggestions are then presented to the user who accepts or rejects them. The acceptance and rejection of a suggestion may influence further suggestions. Further, a conflict checker is used to avoid conflicts introduced by the alignment relationships. The output of the alignment algorithm is a set of alignment relationships between terms from the source ontologies.

To date comparative evaluations of ontology alignment and merge systems have been performed by few groups ([OntoWeb] and [LE03, LT05a, LT05b, LT06]) and only the latter has focused on the quality of the alignment. Further, an ontology alignment contest was held at EON-2004 [Euz04]. The main goal of the contest was to show how ontology alignment tools can be evaluated and a follow-up was planned. An overview of alignment systems and a comparison between different alignment strategies can be found in [LT05a, LT05b, LT06].

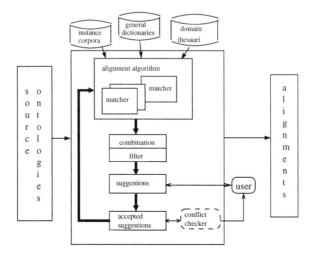

Fig. 1. A general alignment strategy [LT05b]

2.3   SAMBO

SAMBO[1] (System for Aligning and Merging Biomedical Ontologies) is an alignment and merge system for biomedical ontologies developed using the general framework defined in [LT05b]. The current implementation supports ontologies in OWL and DAML+OIL formats. Several kinds of matchers are used [LT05a, LT05b, LT06], including the basic algorithm described in this paper. These matchers can be combined using different weights and a threshold for filtering can be set. For each alignment suggestion the user can decide whether the terms are equivalent, there is an is-a relation between the terms, or the suggestion is rejected (figure 2). At each point in time during the alignment process the user can view the ontologies represented in trees with the information on which actions have been performed, and she can check how many suggestions still need to be processed. In addition to the suggestion mode, the system has a manual mode in which the user can view the ontologies and manually align terms.

3   Alignment Algorithms

In this paper we present algorithms for suggesting alignments between two biomedical ontologies which focus on relationships between concepts. The algorithms make use of life science literature that is related to these concepts. They build on the intuition that a similarity measure between concepts in different ontologies can be computed based on the probability that documents about one concept are also about the other concept and vice versa. We propose a basic algorithm as well as two extensions that take the structure of the ontologies into account.

---

[1] The home page for SAMBO is http://www.ida.liu.se/~iislab/projects/SAMBO/

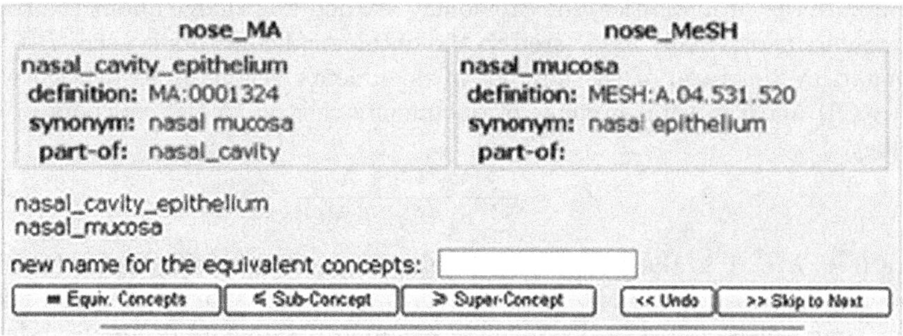

Fig. 2. Alignment suggestion

The algorithms contain the following basic steps.

1. **Generate corpora.** For each ontology that we want to align we generate a corpus of PubMed abstracts. PubMed [PubMed] is a service of the National Library of Medicine that includes over 15 millions citations from MEDLINE [MEDLINE] and other biomedical journals.
2. **Generating the classifiers.** For each ontology a document classifier is generated. This classifier returns for a given document the concept that is most closely related. To generate a classifier the corpus of abstracts associated to the classifier's ontology is used.
3. **Classification.** Documents of one ontology are classified by the document classifier of the other ontology and visa versa.
4. **Calculate similarities.** A similarity measure between concepts in the different ontologies is computed.

In the steps 2 and 3 of our algorithms we use (variants of) the naive Bayes classification algorithm. In the remainder of this section we describe the intuition behind a naive Bayes classifier for classifying text documents with respect to ontological concepts and present the different algorithms in more detail.

3.1   Text Classification Based on Naive Bayes Classifier

A naive Bayes classifier classifies a document d as related to a concept C in an ontology if the highest value for the posterior probability of a concept given the document d is obtained for the concept C. The posterior probability of concept C given document d is estimated using Bayes' rule [Mit97]:

$$P(C|d) = \frac{P(C)P(d|C)}{P(d)}$$

As $P(d)$ is independent of the concepts, it can be ignored. Also, the logarithm of the probability is often computed instead of the actual probability. This gives:

$$logP(C|d) \approx logP(C)P(d|C) = logP(C) + logP(d|C)$$

To evaluate the probabilities, the previously learned knowledge about the training documents originally associated to the ontological concepts is used. $P(C)$ is estimated by the ratio of the number of documents originally associated with C ($n_D(C)$) and the total number of documents related to the concepts in the ontology.

$$P(C) = \frac{n_D(C) + \lambda}{\sum_i n_D(C_i) + \lambda|O|}$$

where $0 < \lambda \leq 1$ is the Laplace smoothing parameter[2], and $|O|$ is the total number of concepts in the ontology. The term $P(d|C)$ is estimated by the probability that words w in the document d occur in documents originally related to C. Assuming that word occurrences are independent of occurrences of other words, we have

$$P(d|C) = \prod_{w \in d} P(w|C)$$

Let $n_W(C, w)$ be the number of occurrences of word w in documents associated with C, and $n_W(C) = \sum_w n_W(C, w)$ be the total number of occurrences of words in documents associated with C. Then $P(w|C)$ is estimated by

$$P(w|C) = \frac{n_W(C, w) + \lambda}{n_W(C) + \lambda|V|}$$

where λ is the earlier defined Laplace smoothing parameter, and $|V|$ is the size of the vocabulary, i.e. the number of distinct words in all of the training documents.

3.2   Basic Algorithm

We now describe the different steps in the basic algorithm in more detail.

1. **Generate corpora.** For each ontology we generate a corpus based on documents that are related to the concepts in the ontology. For each concept we use the concept name as a query term for PubMed and retrieve abstracts of documents that contain the query term in their title or abstract using the programming utilities [SW] provided by the retrieval system Entrez [Entrez]. A maximum number of retrieved abstracts per concept needs to be set beforehand.
2. **Generating the classifiers.** For each ontology a naive Bayes classifier[3] is generated. During the classifier generation $P(C)$ and $P(w|C)$ are calculated for every concept based on the corpus of abstracts associated to the ontology.
3. **Classification.** The naive Bayes classifier for one ontology is applied to every abstract in the abstract corpus of the other ontology and vice versa. For every abstract the classifier calculates $logP(C|d)$ with respect to every concept and classifies the abstract to the concept with the highest value for the posterior probability. The classifier keeps track of how the abstracts associated to concepts in one ontology are distributed over concepts in the other ontology.

---

[2] In the implementation $\lambda = 1$.

[3] The implementation of the naive Bayes classifier is based on the code available at http://www.cs.utexas.edu/users/mooney/ir-course/

4. **Calculate similarities.** As the last step we compute a similarity between concepts in different ontologies. We define the similarity between a concept C_1 from the first ontology and a concept C_2 from the second ontology as:

$$sim(C_1, C_2) = \frac{n_{NBC2}(C_1, C_2) + n_{NBC1}(C_2, C_1)}{n_D(C_1) + n_D(C_2)}$$

where $n_D(C)$ is the number of abstracts originally associated with C, and $n_{NBCx}(C_p, C_q)$ is the number of abstracts associated with C_p that are also related to C_q as found by classifier $NBCx$ related to ontology x.

The pairs of concepts with a similarity measure greater or equal than a predefined threshold are then presented to the user as candidate alignments.

3.3 Structure-Based Extensions of the Basic Algorithm

Most biomedical ontologies are organized using is-a relations. Therefore, the ontologies have inherent information about concepts and sub-concepts and this information could be used during the alignment process. In this section we propose extensions of the basic algorithm that take the structure (is-a relations) of the original ontologies into account by assuming that abstracts that are related to the sub-concepts of a concept C are also related to concept C. The first extension takes the structure into account during the generation of the classifiers. In the second extension we use a different similarity measure.

Structure-based classifier. This algorithm extends the classifier generation step (step 2) of the basic algorithm. To calculate the posterior probability of concept C given document d while taking into account the structure of the classifier's ontology, $P(C)$ and $P(w|C)$ are defined as follows (with $n_D(C)$, $|O|$, λ, $n_W(C, w)$ and $n_W(C)$ as defined before).

$$P(C) = \frac{\sum_{C_j \subseteq C} n_D(C_j) + \lambda}{\sum_i n_D(C_i) + \lambda|O|}, P(w|C) = \frac{\sum_{C_i \subseteq C} n_W(C_i, w) + \lambda}{\sum_{C_i \subseteq C} n_W(C_i) + \lambda|V|}$$

This is equivalent to extending the corpus of documents for each concept C in the ontology by including the documents related to the sub-concepts of the concept C, and then calculating the posterior probabilities using the previously defined naive Bayes classifier.

Structure-based similarity measure. A structure-based similarity between a concept C_1 from the first ontology and a concept C_2 from the second ontology can be defined as (with $n_D(C)$ and $n_{NBCx}(C_p, C_q)$ as defined before):

$$sim_{struct}(C_1, C_2) = \frac{\sum_{C_i \subseteq C_1, C_j \subseteq C_2} n_{NBC2}(C_i, C_j) + \sum_{C_i \subseteq C_1, C_j \subseteq C_2} n_{NBC1}(C_j, C_i)}{\sum_{C_i \subseteq C_1} n_D(C_i) + \sum_{C_j \subseteq C_2} n_D(C_j)}$$

In this definition the similarity between concepts is computed based on the naive Bayes classifiers applied to the concepts and their sub-concepts.

4   Evaluation

In our evaluation we have focused on several aspects. First, we investigated the influence of the number of PubMed abstracts on the quality of the suggestions. Further, we compare the proposed algorithms with respect to the quality of the suggestions they generate and the time they take to generate the suggestions. We also compare them to other matchers implemented in SAMBO with respect to the quality of the suggestions and investigate the combination of the proposed algorithms and the other SAMBO matchers.

4.1   Set-Up

Test cases. In the evaluation we create five cases from several well-known biomedical ontologies. For the first two cases we use a part of a GO ontology [GO00] together with a part of SigO [TNK98]. Each case was chosen in such a way that there is an overlap between the GO part and the SigO part. The first case, *B* (behavior), contains 57 terms from GO and 10 terms from SigO. The second case, *ID* (immune defense), contains 73 terms from GO and 17 terms from SigO. We used more terms from GO than from SigO because the granularity of GO is higher than the granularity of SigO for these topics. The other cases are taken from two biomedical ontologies that are available from OBO [OBO]: MeSH (anatomy category) and MA. The two ontologies cover a similar subject domain, anatomy, and are developed independently. The three cases used in our test are: *nose* (containing 15 terms from MeSH and 18 terms from MA), *ear* (containing 39 terms from MeSH and 77 terms from MA), and *eye* (containing 45 terms from MeSH and 112 terms from MA). We translated the ontologies from the GO flat file format to OWL retaining identifiers, names, synonyms, definitions and is-a and part-of relations. The synonyms were transformed into equivalence statements. Domain experts were asked to analyze the cases and provide alignment relationships based on equivalence and is-a relations. In our evaluations we have used the ontologies and the alignment relationships from the experts as they were provided to us.

Table 1. Number of abstracts

Ontology	concepts	100	90-99	80-89	70-79	60-69	50-59	40-49	30-39	20-29	10-19	1-9	0
B-GO	57	37	0	2	2	2	0	0	0	1	3	4	6
B-SigO	10	10	0	0	0	0	0	0	0	0	0	0	0
ID-GO	73	44	1	2	0	3	0	1	0	3	4	1	14
ID-SigO	17	17	0	0	0	0	0	0	0	0	0	0	0
nose-MA	18	13	0	0	0	1	0	1	0	0	0	3	0
nose-MeSH	15	15	0	0	0	0	0	0	0	0	0	0	0
ear-MA	77	48	1	0	1	3	0	1	2	2	5	9	5
ear-MeSH	39	34	0	1	0	0	0	0	0	1	1	1	1
eye-MA	112	84	2	1	1	3	3	0	1	2	7	8	0
eye-MeSH	45	37	0	0	0	0	2	0	1	1	1	1	2

PubMed. For the generation of the corpora we used PubMed as it was available on October 23, 2005. (All corpora generated between 11.42 and 13.15 CEST.) We generated different corpora for each ontology by assigning a maximum of 20, 40, 60, 80 and 100 PubMed abstracts, respectively, for each concept in the source ontologies. The corpus generated using a maximum of 20 abstracts is a sub-set of the corpus generated using a maximum of 40 abstracts, and similarly for 60, 80 and 100. The retrieval system for PubMed did not always find the allowed number of abstracts for all concepts. Table 1 shows for how many concepts the system retrieved 100, between 90 and 99, ... , between 1-9 and no abstracts. When more abstracts than allowed were found, we retrieved the most recent abstracts, otherwise all abstracts were retrieved. We observe that when the allowed number of abstracts is 100, in some cases only for 60% of the concepts 100 abstracts were retrieved. Even when 20 abstracts were allowed, not for all concepts this number of abstracts was retrieved. In this experiment there is no apparent relationship between the location of a concept in the is-a hierarchy and how many abstracts are retrieved for that concept.

4.2   Evaluation Results

Influence of the number of PubMed abstracts on the quality of the suggestions. In table 2 we present the quality of suggestions generated by the basic algorithm with different numbers of abstracts. The cases are given in the first column. The second column represents the number of expected suggestions provided by domain experts. In our evaluation we consider only expected suggestions related to equivalence of terms or is-a relations between terms. For instance, in the ear case, there are 27 alignments that are specified by domain experts. This is the minimal set of suggestions that matchers are expected to generate for a perfect recall. This set does not include the inferred suggestions. Inferred suggestions are counted neither as correct nor as wrong suggestions. An example of an inferred suggestion is that incus is a kind of ear ossicle. In this case we know that auditory bone (MA) is equivalent to ear ossicle (MeSH), and incus is a kind of auditory bone in MA. Then the system should derive that incus is a kind of ear ossicle. The third column represents the threshold value. Pairs with a similarity value higher than the threshold are suggestions. The other columns present the results. The four numbers in the cells represent the number of suggestions provided by the algorithm, the number of correct suggestions, the number of wrong suggestions and the number of inferred suggestions, respectively. For instance, for the case B with a maximum of 100 PubMed abstracts per concept and threshold 0.4 the algorithm generates 4 suggestions of which 2 suggestions are correct, 1 suggestion is wrong and 1 suggestion is inferred.

For the threshold 0.4 the precision[4] usually becomes higher when the maximum number of abstracts increases, e.g. in the case eye the precision goes up

---

[4] We use precision as it is usually defined in information retrieval, i.e. the number of correct suggestions divided by the number of suggestions. As noted before, inferred suggestions are counted neither correct nor wrong. Similarly, recall is defined as the number of correct suggestions divided by the total number of correct suggestions, in this case the expected suggestions.

Table 2. Influence of number of abstracts. (The cells a/b/c/d represent the number of a) suggestions, b) correct suggestions, c) wrong suggestions and d) inferred suggestions).

Case	ES	Th	20	40	60	80	100
B	4	0.4	3/2/0/1	3/2/1/0	6/2/1/3	4/2/0/2	4/2/1/1
		0.5	2/2/0/0	2/2/0/0	2/2/0/0	2/2/0/0	2/2/0/0
		0.6	2/2/0/0	2/2/0/0	2/2/0/0	2/2/0/0	2/2/0/0
		0.7	2/2/0/0	2/2/0/0	2/2/0/0	2/2/0/0	2/2/0/0
		0.8	2/2/0/0	2/2/0/0	2/2/0/0	2/2/0/0	1/1/0/0
ID	8	0.4	11/4/4/3	9/5/3/1	10/6/3/1	9/6/3/0	9/6/3/0
		0.5	7/4/0/3	6/5/0/1	7/5/1/1	5/5/0/0	5/5/0/0
		0.6	5/4/0/1	4/3/0/1	2/2/0/0	2/2/0/0	2/2/0/0
		0.7	2/2/0/0	1/1/0/0	1/1/0/0	1/1/0/0	1/1/0/0
		0.8	0/0/0/0	0/0/0/0	0/0/0/0	0/0/0/0	0/0/0/0
nose	7	0.4	7/5/2/0	6/5/1/0	6/5/1/0	6/5/1/0	6/5/1/0
		0.5	6/5/1/0	5/5/0/0	6/5/1/0	6/5/1/0	6/5/1/0
		0.6	5/5/0/0	5/5/0/0	5/5/0/0	5/5/0/0	5/5/0/0
		0.7	5/5/0/0	5/5/0/0	5/5/0/0	5/5/0/0	5/5/0/0
		0.8	4/4/0/0	5/5/0/0	3/3/0/0	3/3/0/0	3/3/0/0
ear	27	0.4	20/16/4/0	19/16/3/0	19/16/3/0	18/16/2/0	18/16/2/0
		0.5	18/16/2/0	17/15/2/0	15/14/1/0	15/14/1/0	15/14/1/0
		0.6	14/14/0/0	15/14/1/0	11/10/1/0	12/11/1/0	12/11/1/0
		0.7	11/11/0/0	11/10/1/0	11/10/1/0	11/10/1/0	11/10/1/0
		0.8	5/5/0/0	5/5/0/0	4/4/0/0	3/3/0/0	3/3/0/0
eye	27	0.4	33/19/13/1	32/18/13/1	27/18/9/0	27/19/8/0	25/18/7/0
		0.5	20/17/3/0	20/18/2/0	20/17/3/0	18/16/2/0	18/17/1/0
		0.6	16/16/0/0	17/16/1/0	15/14/1/0	14/14/0/0	14/14/0/0
		0.7	12/12/0/0	11/11/0/0	13/13/0/0	11/11/0/0	10/10/0/0
		0.8	5/5/0/0	5/5/0/0	5/5/0/0	5/5/0/0	3/3/0/0

from 0.575 to 0.72. The exception is the case B where we obtain the best result when the maximum number of abstracts is 20 or 40. As the maximum number of abstracts increases, no more correct suggestions are found, except in the ID case where two more correct *is-a* relationships are found when the maximum number of abstracts is higher than 40. For higher threshold values the number of suggestions diminishes, e.g. in the ID case where the number of suggestions goes down to 0 and both correct and wrong suggestions are filtered out. When the maximum number of abstracts increases, the number of correct suggestions goes down even faster when the threshold becomes higher. The results of this experiment suggest that the quality of the suggestions does not necessarily become better when we have larger corpora of abstracts. The experiment also shows that the corpora have an impact on the quality of the suggestions.

Quality of the suggestions. In table 3 we compare the quality of the suggestions generated by our basic (Basic) algorithm, the extension that takes the structure into account during the generation of the classifier (StrucCl), the ex-

Table 3. Comparison of matchers: quality of the suggestions

Case	ES	Th	Basic	StrucCl	StrucSim	StrucClSim
B	4	0.4	4/2/1/1	5/2/0/3	20/3/6/11	7/1/0/6
		0.5	2/2/0/0	3/2/0/1	7/1/2/4	5/1/0/4
		0.6	2/2/0/0	2/2/0/0	5/1/0/4	4/0/0/4
		0.7	2/2/0/0	1/1/0/0	3/1/0/2	2/0/0/2
		0.8	1/1/0/0	0/0/0/0	2/0/0/2	1/0/0/1
ID	8	0.4	9/6/3/0	4/3/0/1	14/6/4/4	5/2/1/2
		0.5	5/5/0/0	2/2/0/0	9/5/2/2	4/1/1/2
		0.6	2/2/0/0	0/0/0/0	5/2/1/2	4/1/1/2
		0.7	1/1/0/0	0/0/0/0	4/1/1/2	4/1/1/2
		0.8	0/0/0/0	0/0/0/0	4/1/1/2	3/0/1/2
nose	7	0.4	6/5/1/0	7/5/2/0	9/5/2/2	8/5/2/1
		0.5	6/5/1/0	5/5/0/0	6/4/1/1	4/3/0/1
		0.6	5/5/0/0	5/5/0/0	4/3/0/1	3/3/0/0
		0.7	5/5/0/0	2/2/0/0	3/3/0/0	1/1/0/0
		0.8	3/3/0/0	2/2/0/0	1/1/0/0	1/1/0/0
ear	27	0.4	18/16/2/0	15/11/2/2	24/12/4/8	14/8/3/3
		0.5	15/14/1/0	6/5/0/1	16/11/1/4	5/4/0/1
		0.6	12/11/1/0	3/3/0/0	12/10/1/1	1/1/0/0
		0.7	11/10/1/0	1/1/0/0	10/9/1/0	0/0/0/0
		0.8	3/3/0/0	1/1/0/0	2/2/0/0	0/0/0/0
eye	27	0.4	25/18/7/0	25/11/11/3	34/14/15/5	16/8/6/2
		0.5	18/17/1/0	8/7/1/0	21/12/6/3	10/4/4/2
		0.6	14/14/0/0	3/3/0/0	14/9/4/1	1/0/1/0
		0.7	10/10/0/0	1/1/0/0	9/7/2/0	1/0/1/0
		0.8	3/3/0/0	1/1/0/0	3/3/0/0	0/0/0/0

tension that uses the structure-based similarity measure (StrucSim) and an algorithm using both extensions (StrucClSim). In the evaluation we generated corpora for each ontology by assigning a maximum of 100 PubMed abstracts for each concept in the source ontologies.

In most of the cases Basic outperforms the structure-based algorithms. Only in very few cases the structure-based algorithms showed higher precision and recall. For the B, ID, and some settings of the nose, ear and eye cases, StrucSim returns the largest number of suggestions. A large part of these suggestions are inferred or wrong. The lowest number of suggestions is returned by StrucCl and StrucClSim. Among the structure-based algorithms, StrucSim generates the largest number of correct suggestions for the ID, ear and eye cases. In some cases of B and nose, StrucSim is outperformed by StrucCl. The only new correct suggestion is found by StrucSim and StrClSim for the ear case with the threshold 0.5 - (auditory bone, ear ossicle). The concepts in the suggestion have common sub-concepts. For the structure-based algorithms we noted that the similarity value for a pair of concepts depends to a large degree on the content of the abstracts related to the sub-concepts of the concepts in the suggestion (StrucCl, StrucClSim) and on how the abstracts of one ontology are classified by the classifier of the other ontology (StrucSim, StrucClSim). This dependency is the source of improved results in some of the test cases, but it may also result in the decreased quality of the results.

The results of StrucCl illustrated that the use of the abstracts of sub-concepts may cause both positive and negative results. Some of the wrong suggestions were removed based on the fact that abstracts related to sub-concepts dealt with unrelated topics. For instance, (circadian rhythm, sleep response) in B gets a lower similarity value in StrucCl than in Basic. However, at the same time new wrong suggestions were introduced. For instance, (reproductive behavior, feeding behavior) is a wrong suggestion for B. In this case abstracts related to their sub-concepts are about behavior. Also, some of the correct suggestions were removed by the algorithm. In some of these cases the abstracts of the sub-concepts included many more non-relevant concepts or very little relevant concepts, which caused a decrease in probabilities for the important terms in the abstracts. Some of the correct suggestions were removed because a number of abstracts classified to certain concepts by Basic were classified to other concepts by StrucCl.

Many of the suggestions generated by StrucSim are inferred suggestions, which illustrates the fact that sub-concepts may give strong support for the analyzed concepts. However, they may also be the cause of wrong suggestions.

For instance, (defense response, body level function) is a wrong suggestion in the ID case and both concepts have immune response as their sub-concept. In our algorithms we did not propagate the abstracts via part-of. This caused several wrong suggestions in the MA-MeSH cases as part-of and is-a are used differently in the two ontologies.

StrucSimCl combines the StrucCl and StrucSim approaches. In none of the cases StrucSimCl returned higher similarity values for the correct suggestions than the other two structure-based algorithms. We observed that low similarity values of StrucCl or StrucSim have a large influence on the final similarity. In a number of cases StrucClSim returns low similarity values even though StrucCl and StrucSim return high similarities when executed separately. The poor performance of the algorithm could be explained by the fact that an abstract can be classified to only one concept. In some cases this results in abstracts previously classified to a concept to be classified to a super-concept.

Some expected suggestions were not found by any of our instance-based algorithms. One reason could be the low number of abstracts in the generated corpora for some concepts. For instance, in the eye case, (macula, macula lutea) is not returned, where macula lutea has only 26 related abstracts. Also, the abstracts in the corpora may cover different domains.

Performance of the algorithms. We also evaluated the time it takes for the discussed algorithms to compute the suggestions. For all of the algorithms we generated the PubMed corpora beforehand. The time for loading the ontologies ranges from 0.9 to 3.2 seconds. In most of the cases the time is around 1.5 seconds. In table 4 we present the time to generate suggestions. This covers the time for learning the classifier and the time for computing the similarity values. In the nose case, where a small number of abstracts is classified and the

Table 4. Comparison of matchers: time for computation of the suggestions (in seconds)

Case	Basic	StrucCl	StrucSim	StrucClSim
B	421.2	567.3	497.8	570.4
ID	354.1	824.2	603.0	1001.0
nose	216.1	219.1	213.1	223.3
ear	667.5	1097.1	904.5	1032.5
eye	1848.1	2012.5	1982.5	2024.8

ontologies contain only few is-a relations, there is no significant difference in the performance of the algorithms. For larger cases there is a tendency that there is an increase of time from Basic to StrucSim to StrucCl to StrucClSim. We used a SUN Ultra 5_10 Sparc workstation for these tests.

Quality of the suggestions compared to other algorithms. In table 5 we show the quality of the suggestions of other matchers that were presented in [LT06] (preliminary results in [LT05b]): a terminological matcher (Term), a terminological matcher using WordNet (TermWN), and a matcher (Dom) using

Table 5. Other matchers: quality of the suggestions [LT06]

Case	ES	Th	Term	TermWN	Dom
B	4	0.4	58/4/22/32	58/4/22/32	4/4/0/0
		0.5	35/4/13/18	35/4/13/18	4/4/0/0
		0.6	13/4/4/5	13/4/4/5	4/4/0/0
		0.7	6/4/0/2	6/4/0/2	4/4/0/0
		0.8	4/4/0/0	4/4/0/0	4/4/0/0
ID	8	0.4	96/7/66/23	96/7/66/23	4/4/0/0
		0.5	49/7/25/17	49/7/25/17	4/4/0/0
		0.6	15/5/4/6	16/5/5/6	4/4/0/0
		0.7	7/5/2/0	7/5/2/0	4/4/0/0
		0.8	6/4/0/2	6/4/0/2	4/4/0/0
nose	7	0.4	47/7/36/4	48/7/37/4	7/7/0/0
		0.5	27/7/17/3	28/7/18/3	7/7/0/0
		0.6	7/6/1/0	8/6/2/0	7/7/0/0
		0.7	6/6/0/0	6/6/0/0	6/6/0/0
		0.8	6/6/0/0	6/6/0/0	6/6/0/0
ear	27	0.4	147/26/104/17	155/26/110/19	26/23/2/1
		0.5	92/26/58/8	99/26/65/8	26/23/2/1
		0.6	47/26/19/2	47/26/19/2	26/23/2/1
		0.7	33/25/8/0	34/26/8/0	24/22/2/0
		0.8	26/24/2/0	28/25/3/0	24/22/2/0
eye	27	0.4	130/26/95/9	135/26/100/9	22/21/1/0
		0.5	72/23/42/7	74/23/44/7	22/21/1/0
		0.6	33/22/10/1	33/22/10/1	22/21/1/0
		0.7	24/21/3/0	24/21/3/0	19/18/1/0
		0.8	19/18/1/0	22/20/2/0	19/18/1/0

domain knowledge in the form of the Unified Medical Language System (UMLS) of the U.S. National Library of Medicine [UMLS]. The terminological matcher contains matching algorithms based on the names and synonyms of concepts and relations. The matcher is a combination matcher based on two approximate string matching algorithms (n-gram and edit distance) and a linguistic algorithm. In TermWN a general thesaurus, WordNet [WordNet], is used to enhance the similarity measure by using the hypernym relationships in WordNet. Dom uses the Metathesaurus in the UMLS which contains more than 100 biomedical and health-related vocabularies. The Metathesaurus is organized using concepts. The concepts may have synonyms which are the terms in the different vocabularies in the Metathesaurus that have the same intended meaning. The similarity of two terms in the source ontologies is determined by their relationship in UMLS. For more detailed information about these matchers we refer to [LT06].

We compare these matchers with Basic. The quality of the suggestions for Basic varies in the different ontologies in this evaluation. In the ID case it produces the best result among the matchers. It avoids the wrong suggestions with slightly different names, such as (B cell activation, T Cell Activation). It also finds the suggestion (natural killer cell activation, Natural Killer Cell Response), which is not found by Dom. However, in the eye case it produces the worst result. In this case all its correct suggestions are also found by the other matchers. We also note that the other matchers take synonyms into account and as our test ontologies contain many synonyms, their results improve considerably.

Combination with other matchers. Table 6 presents the quality of the suggestions considering the combination of the different matchers. The suggestions are determined based on the combination of the similarity values measured by individual matchers using weights, $sim(C_1, C_2) = (\sum_{k=1}^{n} w_k * sim_k(C_1, C_2))/\sum_{k=1}^{n} w_k$, where sim_k and w_k represent the similarity values and weights, respectively, for the different matchers. In the experiment we used 1 as the weight for each matcher and 0.5 as the threshold value. The combination of our instance-based algorithms with Dom and TermWN leads to higher quality results. For the B, nose and ear cases, the instance-based algorithms combined with Dom return the same num-

Table 6. Combination of matchers

Case	ES	Matcher	Basic	StrucCl	StrucSim	StrucClSim
B	4	TermWN	6/4/0/2	5/4/0/1	10/4/2/4	6/4/0/2
		Dom	4/4/0/0	4/4/0/0	4/4/0/0	4/4/0/0
ID	8	TermWN	8/7/1/0	5/4/0/1	12/7/2/3	7/5/1/1
		Dom	4/4/0/0	4/4/0/0	4/4/0/0	4/4/0/0
nose	7	TermWN	8/7/1/0	8/7/1/0	10/7/2/1	8/7/1/0
		Dom	7/7/0/0	7/7/0/0	7/7/0/0	7/7/0/0
ear	27	TermWN	27/22/5/0	26/22/4/0	28/22/5/1	28/22/5/1
		Dom	24/22/2/0	24/22/2/0	24/22/2/0	24/22/2/0
eye	27	TermWN	24/21/3/0	23/19/4/0	30/21/8/1	21/19/2/0
		Dom	20/19/1/0	19/18/1/0	20/19/1/0	19/18/1/0

ber of correct suggestions as in the combination with TermWN. For the ID and eye cases the combination with TermWN gives better recall but lower precision. Dom tends to remove suggestions for which it finds no relationship in its domain knowledge. As could be expected from the results in table 3, StrucSim combined with TermWN returns more correct suggestions than StrucCl combined with TermWN at the expense of a larger number of wrong suggestions. All correct suggestions that are found by the combinations of matchers were also found by TermWN. The combinations of TermWN and Dom with the instance-based algorithms remove some of the wrong and inferred suggestions. In particular, for TermWN a large number of redundant suggestions were eliminated in the combination. However, at the same time some correct suggestions returned by TermWN and Dom were removed in the combination.

5   Related Work

Some ontology alignment and merging systems provide alignment strategies using literature, such as ArtGen [MW02], FCA-Merge [SM01] and OntoMapper [SYT02]. The basic alignment algorithm in ArtGen calculates the similarity between concepts based on their names which are seen as lists of words. One method to compute the similarity between a pair of words is based on the similarity between the contexts (1000-character neighborhoods) of all occurrences of the words in a set of domain-specific Web pages. In FCA-Merge the user constructs a merged ontology based on a concept lattice. The concept lattice is derived using formal concept analysis based on how documents from a given domain-specific corpus are classified to the concepts in the ontologies using natural language processing techniques. OntoMapper provides an ontology alignment algorithm using Bayesian learning. A set of documents (abstracts of technical papers taken from ACM's digital library and Citeseer) is assigned to each concept in the ontologies. Two raw similarity scores matrices for the ontologies are computed by the Rainbow text classifier. The similarity between the concepts is calculated based on these two matrices using the Bayesian method.

There are systems that implement alignment algorithms based on the structure of the ontologies. Most systems rely on the existence of previously aligned concepts. For instance, Anchor-PROMPT [NM01] determines the similarity of concepts by the frequency of their appearance along the paths between previously aligned concepts. The paths may be composed of any kind of relations. Also SAMBO as described in [LT05b] provides such a component where the similarity between concepts is augmented based on their location in the is-a hierarchy relative to already aligned concepts. However, for our test ontologies, these methods often did not perform well. In this paper we proposed methods that do not require previously aligned concepts. Also OntoMapper does not require previously aligned concepts and takes the documents from the sub-concepts into account when computing the similarity between two concepts. However, as this is hardcoded in the method, it is not clear how the structure of the ontologies influences the result of the computation.

6   Conclusion

In this paper we proposed and experimented with instance-based alignment strategies that use life science literature for aligning biomedical ontologies. We proposed a basic algorithm as well as extensions that take the structure of the ontologies into account. We evaluated the influence of the size of the literature corpus, the quality and performance of the strategies and their combination with other strategies. The basic algorithm outperforms the structure-based strategies in most cases, although compared to the other matchers in SAMBO the quality of the suggestions varies for the different cases. In some cases it produces the best result, in some cases the worst. An advantage of our structure-based strategies is that they can be used without information about previously aligned concepts, as many other systems require. However, the best results are obtained when the instance-based strategies are combined with other strategies. The other strategies usually provide new correct suggestions while the instance-based algorithms usually have the effect of removing wrong suggestions.

There are a number of issues that we still want to investigate. A limitation of our algorithms is that abstracts are only classified to one concept. We want to extend our strategies by allowing abstracts to be classified to 0, 1 or more concepts. We are also interested in looking at other classification algorithms. Regarding the structure the ontologies in the current experiments are reasonably simple taxonomies. We want to investigate whether the structure-based strategies lead to similar results for other types of ontologies. Further, our matchers could be enhanced to use synonyms and domain knowledge.

References

[CGGG03]   Collins F, Green E, Guttmacher A, Guyer M (2003) A vision for the future of genomics research. *Nature*, 422: 835-847.

[Entrez]   Entrez. http://www.ncbi.nlm.nih.gov/Database/index.html

[Euz04]   Euzenat J (2004) Introduction to the EON ontology alignment context. *3rd Int. Workshop on the Evaluation of Ontology-based Tools.*

[GO00]   The Gene Ontology Consortium (2000) Gene Ontology: tool for the unification of biology. *Nature Genetics*, 25(1):25-29. http://www.geneontology.org/.

[Gom99]   Gómez-Pérez A (1999) Ontological Engineering: A state of the Art. *Expert Update*, 2(3):33-43.

[JL05]   Jakoniene V, Lambrix P (2005) Ontology-based Integration for Bioinformatics. *VLDB Workshop on Ontologies-based techniques for DataBases and Information Systems - ODBIS 2005*, pp 55-58.

[Lam04]   Lambrix P (2004) Ontologies in Bioinformatics and Systems Biology. Chapter 8 in Dubitzky W, Azuaje F (eds) *Artificial Intelligence Methods and Tools for Systems Biology*, pp 129-146, Springer. ISBN: 1-4020-2859-8.

[Lam05]   Lambrix P (2005) Towards a Semantic Web for Bioinformatics using Ontology-based Annotation. *14th IEEE WET-ICE*, pp 3-7. Invited talk.

[LE03]   Lambrix P, Edberg A (2003) Evaluation of ontology merging tools in bioinformatics. *Pacific Symposium on Biocomputing*, 8:589-600.

[LT05a]   Lambrix P, Tan H, (2005) Merging DAML+OIL Ontologies. Barzdins, Caplinskas (eds) *Databases and Information Systems*, pp 249-258, IOS Press.

[LT05b]   Lambrix P, Tan H (2005) A Framework for Aligning Ontologies. *3rd Workshop on Principles and Practice of Semantic Web Reasoning*, LNCS 3703, pp 17-31.

[LT06]   Lambrix P, Tan H (2005) SAMBO - a System for Aligning and Merging Biomedical Ontologies. Submitted.

[MEDLINE]   MEDLINE.   http://www.nlm.nih.gov/databases/databases_medline. html

[Mit97]   Mitchell T (1997) *Machine Learning*. McGraw-Hill.

[MW02]   Mitra P, Wiederhold G (2002) Resolving terminological heterogeneity in ontologies. *ECAI Workshop on Ontologies and Semantic Interoperability*.

[NM01]   Noy N, Musen M (2001) Anchor-PROMPT: Using Non-Local Context for Semantic Matching. *IJCAI Workshop on Ontologies and Information Sharing*, pp 63-70.

[OBO]   Open Biomedical Ontologies. http://obo.sourceforge.net/

[OntoWeb]   OntoWeb Consortium (2002) Deliverables 1.3 (A survey on ontology tools) and 1.4 (A survey on methodologies for developing, maintaining, evaluating and reengineering ontologies).

[Protege]   Protégé. http://protege.stanford.edu/index.html

[PubMed]   PubMed. http://www.ncbi.nlm.nih.gov/entrez/query.fcgi

[REWERSE]   REWERSE. http://www.rewerse.net

[SM01]   Stumme G, Mädche A (2001) FCA-Merge: Bottom-up merging of ontologies. *17th IJCAI*, pp 225-230.

[SW]   Sayers E, Wheeler D. Building Customized Data Pipelines Using the Entrez Programming Utilities (eUtils). *NCBI Coursework*.

[SYT02]   Sushama S, Yun P, Timothy F (2002) Using Explicit Information To Map Between Two Ontologies. *AAMAS Workshop on Ontologies in Agent Systems*.

[TNK98]   Takai-Igarashi T, Nadaoka Y, Kaminuma T (1998) A Database for Cell Signaling Networks. *Journal of Computational Biology* 5(4):747-754.

[UMLS]   UMLS. http://www.nlm.nih.gov/research/umls/

[WordNet]   WordNet. http://wordnet.princeton.edu/

Improving Literature Preselection
by Searching for Images

Brigitte Mathiak[1], Andreas Kupfer[1], Richard Münch[2],
Claudia Täubner[1], and Silke Eckstein[1]

[1] Institut für Informationssysteme, TU Braunschweig, Germany
{b.mathiak, a.kupfer, c.taeubner, s.eckstein}@tu-bs.de
[2] Institut für Mikrobiologie, TU Braunschweig, Germany
r.muench@tu-bs.de

Abstract. In this paper we present a picture search engine for life science literature and show how it can be used to improve literature preselection. This preselection is needed as a way to compensate for the vast amounts of literature that are available. While searching for DNA binding sites for example, we wanted to add the results of specific experiments (DNAse I footprint and EMSA) to our database. The preselection via abstract search was very unspecific (150 000 hits), but by looking for paper with images concerning the experiments, we could improve precision immensely. They are displayed like hits in a search engine, allowing easy and quick quality assessment without having to read through the whole paper. The images are found by their annotation in the paper: the figure caption. To identify that, we analyse the layout of the paper: the position of the image and the surrounding text.

1 Introduction

Preselection is a necessary step in literature annotation, to cope with the large amounts of literature available. The literature is selected to cover topics of interest, the more specific the better, so less paper have to be read. Preselection is usually done by keyword search on abstracts eg. via the search engine on PubMed [1].

The PRODORIC database [2] contains very special data like DNA binding sites of prokaryotic transcriptional regulators. This data is generated via specific experiments like DNAse I footprints or ElectroMobility gel Shift Assays (EMSA) that are generally not mentioned in the abstracts of scientific literature. The search for general key words classifying this comprehensive field like "gene regulation", "promoter" or "binding site" results in over 150,000 hits, and even with additional refinement only 10-20% contain appropriate data. Therefore it is necessary to screen all the hits manually to obtain literature references suitable for database annotation. Of these, those are especially valuable that contain pictures of the DNAse I footprint or EMSA assay, because they represent verified information of high quality. This quality assessment can be important on further exploration of the subject.

The special problem posed by this experimental data, is that keywords searches in abstracts or even full text are ambiguous. The experimental procedures are rarely mentioned in the abstract and in the full text, experimental methods belonging to the overall

E.G. Bremer et al. (Eds.): KDLL 2006, LNBI 3886, pp. 18–28, 2006.

topic are often referenced eg. in literature overview. By using the figure captions we can accurately find pictures for each experiment.

It has already been shown that some of the defining information of a publication is not mentioned in the abstract. Obviously, more information can be obtained by searching through full text paper [3], though precision has decreased. In [4], a competition in literature annotation, it has been observed that analyzing the figure caption is of great value to improve the precision. Classifying the different sections of a paper to analyse them seperately has been successfully attempted in [5], but curiously, the figure captions have not been examined in this study.

A scientific document is more complex than it seems. Readers can easily deduce structure and semantics of the different characters and pictures on a page. But most of this structure information is not stored and available when accessing the publication as PDF, without the competence of a human reader.

The basic problem of handling PDFs is that the text information is not freely available. While an HTML file stripped of its tags usually delivers legible text, even the simple task of text extraction from a PDF is rather complicated. Down to the basics, PDF is foremost a visual medium, describing for each glyph (= character or picture) where it should be printed on the page [6]. Most PDF converters simply emulate this glyph-by-glyph positioning in ASCII, HTML or any other formats [7], but information about reading order and overall semantic connection of the text is lost. Still, since the position of all glyphs is known, the original layout can be deduced and the semantical connection can be restored.

For HTML, the layout information has successfully been used to improve the classification of web pages [8]. We extract the same layout information for PDF documents. To prove the viability of our approach, we used the layout information to implement a special search for PDF embedded pictures in scientific publications. Since the figure captions contain much information about the figure, we implemented a search engine, similar to Google Images, to find images not in regular HTML web pages, but in PDFs. We use layout information to associate the picture with the caption. So, if the user wishes to find pictures containing UML-diagramms, he can just enter "UML" to find what he needs.

The paper starts by giving a general overview over the technology used. In section 2, we demonstrate the general workflow of the search engine. Section 3 gives more details about the internal PDF structure. Section 4 describes how the text is put into PDF and how it can be extracted again, while maintaining the layout information. In section 5 we explain the same process for images and section 6 describes image and text coming together as figure and caption. Section 7 finally contains the results we had in our evaluation with the biological data. In the last section we draw some conclusions and discuss further improvements on our search engine.

2   CaptionSearch

We start with a simple technical overview of how the picture search engine works. The process consists of 6 steps from the download to the actual query execution (see Fig. 2), all of them are currently implemented in Java.

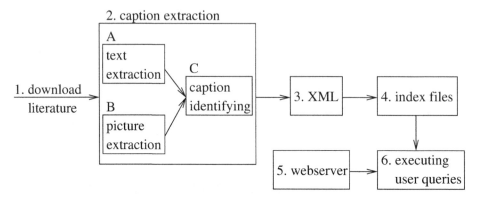

Fig. 1. Overview of the CaptionSearch dataflow

Step 1 is straightforward downloading any kind of literature that might be interesting into a file pool. The technical details of step 2 were mainly already given before. In order to allow for future extensions, we split the process into three parts. Part A works like any PDF to text converter and in fact is based on the Java converter PDFBox [9]. We did a few changes, like refining the coordinate calculations and changing the space detection algorithm. We also keep a lot of the meta-information that is usually lost in the process, like the bounding boxes of all the text blocks, the fonts and font sizes. That information could also be used by a different algorithm.

Part B extracts the pictures into files and adds fake picture text blocks that contain information on the position of the picture and the filename as a link. In part C we perform the algorithm outlined in section 6 to get pairs of picture blocks and text blocks for each pdf.

In step 3 these pairs are written to an xml file (see example below).

```
1 <?xml version="1.0"
                encoding="iso-8859-2"?>
2 <pdf src="10094677.pdf">
3    <img src="pics/10094677.Im4.jpg">
4       <caption>FIG. 4. DNase I
                footprint analysis of ...
5 </caption></img></pdf>
```

Each publication is represented by one file containing a PDF element (line 2-5), which may contain many image elements (like the one in line 3-5), which have the link to the picture as an attribute (line 3) and the caption as a further element (line 4-5).

In Step 4 we use the Digester package [10] to extract the information from the xml files into the indexer. For each figure a virtual document is put into the indexer containing the figure caption to be indexed and the image link and pdf link as metainformation. For the indexing itself, we use the Lucene package [11], which offers fast, Java-based indexing, but also some additional functionality, like a built-in query parser and several so-called analyser that allow us to vary how exactly the captions are indexed and what defines a term.

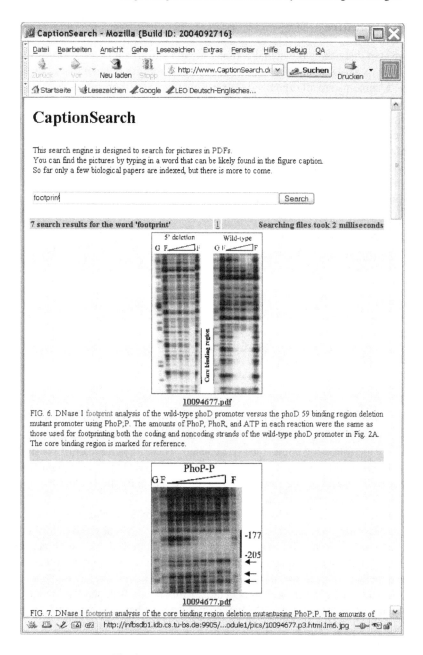

Fig. 2. A screenshot from our search engine

For step 5 we set up a Tomcat webserver [12], using Java servlets [13] to produce the website and to present the query results. In step 6, all queries are executed by a servlet that uses Lucene to fetch the results from the index files and builds a new web page to display the results according to the pre-selected schema.

3 PDF Structure

Before we start discussing the actual text and picture extraction in the sections 4 and 5, we first have to explain some basics about PDF and how its raw data structure works like. PDF documents are all organized the same way: a header, objects and a trailer. The header contains information about the PDF version. The trailer is a bit more complicated containing structural information such as the length of the document, a reference to the root object, and more. Everything else like text information, fonts, images and structuring information is encoded into objects. The two objects (see example below) are structured into an object designation (line 1 and 9), that gives the number the object can be referenced with and object data. Line numbers are included for readability. The data is often proceeded by a dictionary (lines 2-4) that gives additional information about the data.

```
1  1 0 obj
2  << /Length 2 0 R
3     /Filter /FlateDecode
4  >>
5  stream
6  inserted here are 108 bytes of data
7  endstream endobj
8
9  2 0 obj
10   108
11 endobj
```

In line 2 the length of the stream is determined by referencing the second object with the ID 2 0 in line 9 that contains 108 as its data (line 10). In line 3 information is given on how the following stream can be decoded. There are a number of possibilities, FlateDecode is the most common and identical to ZIP [14]. The semantics of the decoded stream depend on the function of the object given by the context the object is referenced in or given explicitly in the dictionary.

The overall structure of the document is mostly hierarchical. The root object, which is given in the trailer, references a pages container object, which references the pages and so on. Mutual information may be shared by referencing the same object several times. The objects are all readable from all objects and may not contain other objects only reference them. Hencefore, the order of the objects does not matter, as all are treated in the same way. The number of objects in the document varies depending on the way it was produced: an average 5 pages document may contain between 20 and 300 objects.

4 Text in PDF

When looking for captions, we first have to analyse all the text that is on the page. For that, we have to take the page object (like the one in the example before) and decode the text stream (the binary code in line 6), the result is a chain of commands that describes the text to be written on that page. The above example shows a short sample taken from a real PDF:

```
1  BT
2  8 0 0 8 52 757.35 Tm
3  /F2 1 Tf
4  0 -1.706 TD
5  (page 354)Tj
6  T*
7  [ (J) -27 (OURN) 27 (AL) -378 (1) ]TJ
8  ET
```

By convention, the parameters of a command are written before the command and all commands are abbreviated to two letters. All text-related commands are between a BT (line 1) and an ET (line 8) which stands for Begin Text and End Text, respectively.

There are 3 different matrices that keep track of the current writing position. The matrices are given as 6 values, like the values in line 2. The first four represent a rotation matrix. The rotation matrix can be used to write landscape text or up-side-down. Also it gives scaling parameters, which are multiplied with the actual fontsizes. The next 2 values give the position on the paper in pixels. The matrix that is set in line 2 with the Tm (set Text matrix) command is the text matrix. The other two matrices are the transformation matrix, which can be set outside the BT-ET environment to move whole text passages and the CTM (Current Transformation Matrix) that is supposed to keep track of the beginning of the line to enable carriage return.

The font size can be set either by the scaling of the matrix or directly when setting the font. The command Tf (see line 3) has two parameters, first the font object, here referenced by name, and the font size. Although the font size is set to 1pt the matrix scales it up to 8pt. In the next line line spacing is defined in text matrix coordinate system, the next line is supposed to start 1.706 times the current font size below the start of the current line. There are also possibilities to define word spacing and character spacing.

In line 5 at last text is written to the screen. The Tj command has a string parameter. Strings are denoted by the brackets around them. The text is now written, using the current matrices and the chosen font. The T* in line 6 marks a carriage return. The text matrix is set to the CTM that stored the coordinates from the beginning of the line. Then the line padding operation as defined in line 4 is executed and the CTM is set to this new coordinates.

In line 7 the second line of text is written. The TJ command, opposing to the Tj command, allows ligatures inside the string. The numbers between the strings modify the horizontal space between the letters. Contra-intuitively, positive numbers mean less space, while negative numbers mean more space. A very large negative number, like the -378 in the example can even be used to produce a space between the words without using the space literal. Since every kind of movement can be such an implicit space or carriage return, we need some algorithm to decide which one is which.

For indexing purposes it is vital to identify correct word borders, otherwise terms may be glued together or torn apart. In those cases it is not possible to find the terms anymore. Unfortunately, the spaces are sometimes not given directly, but instead the characters are just a little more apart from each other than usual. The problem sharpens as theoretically all characters can be written in any kind of order by jumping around with explicitly set coordinates.

In order to identify the spaces anyway, our first run through the text stream just extracts the characters one by one and calculates their bounding boxes. Then the difference vector x_{diff} between two adjacent characters is calculated and rotated in writing direction $\mathbf{R}$.

$$rotationmatrix\ \mathbf{R} =$$

$$\begin{pmatrix} x_{old,\ right} - x_{old,\ left} & y_{old,\ right} - y_{old,\ left} \\ -y_{old,\ right} + y_{old,\ left} & x_{old,\ right} - x_{old,\ left} \end{pmatrix}$$

$$x_{diff} = (x_{new,\ left} - x_{old,\ right}) \frac{\mathbf{R}}{|\mathbf{R}|}$$

The resulting vector is compared to the current modified font size to determine whether this is a space, no space, carriage return or a new block of text. Next, the blocks are sorted and go through a similar procedure. This way the initial information about the order is conserved best.

The blocks bounding boxes are conserved to allow further investigation of their layout, also all changes in fonts or font size and all lines are denoted with their own bounding boxes.

Additional problems which arise are: text overlaps, when e.g. a special font is used to write the accent over à that overlaps the original a and the overall handling of non-identifiable fonts and fonts that give wrong bounding boxes.

5   Images in PDF

Since we want to present the picture along side with the caption, we need to do two things: firstly, we have to know where the image is and secondly, we have to extract the image into a standard readable image format.

The images themselves are stored in so called XObjects. From the text stream an XObject can be called by using the command Do (execute the named XObject).

```
1   22 0 obj
2   << /Type /XObject
3   /Subtype /Image
4   /Name /Im3
5   /Width 580
6   /Height 651
7   /BitsPerComponent 8
8   /ColorSpace /DeviceGray
9   /Length 31853
10  /Filter /DCTDecode>>
11  stream ... endstream endobj
```

This example object represents an image that can be called by entering Im3 Do into the text stream. What happens then is that the object called Im3 is identified and executed. From the object dictionary, we can gain some information like width (line 5) and height (line 6), although this information might not be acurate. The true hight and width are calculated and give, together with the current position the bounding box of the picture.

To actually extract the picture, we need the filter (as given in line 10), in this case DCTDecode, which is the PDF name for Jpeg encoding [15]. The stream simply contains the a jpg-file that can be copied out without further modifications.

Aside from this case, there are a number of possible complications. Natively, all images are given as raster images, like a BitMap. Width and height are given to determine the dimensioning of the raster, BitsPerComponent (see line 7) give the color depth. The Colorspace (given in line 8) maps the colors to the RGB values they are painted in. For filters, there are a number to chose from, some of those are quite old and unfortunately not all have open source libraries to convert them to more publicly known formats. Also it is possible for an image to consist of drawing instructions in the PDF text stream language or they can be inserted in PostScript language.

Since a relatively high number of pictures can not be extracted easily, our next idea is to use a third-party application to extract the pictures seperately. We would then try to match the coordinates given by the program with coordinates of our own. Unfortunately, this is still in prototype phase.

6   Finding the Caption

What we have at this point is the converted text (see section 4), together with its bounding boxes and the pictures with their bounding boxes (see section 5). The next step is to find out which text belongs to which picture.

To achieve this, every text block is weighted according to 2 factors: y_{diff}, the y-proximity in pixels from the bottom line of the picture and x_{diff}, the x-proximity from the left border of the picture. The weighs were chosen by try-and-error. The following formula produced no avoidable errors in the test set.

$$\text{weight } \omega = 10y_{diff} + x_{diff}$$

In order to find captions that are next to the figure or above it, we also introduced a semantic criterium. Figure captions do traditionally begin with "Figure 1:" or something similar. The block that we found with the method described above, is first checked whether or not it has such a denotation. If not, we look at the other blocks in proximity and check them. If there is no "Figure"-block to be found, we stick with the block right below. This is the case, for example, when the caption is prefaced with a filler (dots or a special symbol), or when the image is not scientifical, like for example a logo.

Finding the end of the caption is much less deterministic. Fortunately, most captions have a significant gap before the main text begins again. Also, normally captions are single-column even if the text is two-column. Although we do keep track of the font and the captions are usually written in another font, we do not use this information, since there are just too many publications, that do use the same font and font size for both purposes. Instead we keep strictly to the layout information on where an untypical large gap between line is.

7   Results

In the last few years, the number of biological databases has grown exponentially, from 548 in January 2004 to 719 in January 2005 [16]. Yet, one of the most time-consuming tasks when setting up new databases is the annotation of literature. This time is supposed to be minimized by a suitable preselection. There already exist a number of very interesting search engines. Via PubMed [1], for example, most of the recently written abstracts in life science can be searched. Unfortunately, abstracts often do not mention the exact methods that were used, so for databases that contain experimental data, like the PRODORIC database [2], literature annotation becomes the proverbial search for the needle in the haystack.

Out of 188 papers that were known to contain information about DNA binding sites, 170 did contain extractable pictures. All in all there were 1416 pictures in the PDFs of which 586 could not be extracted using our algorithm from section 5, but since we could identify their position, we indexed the caption anyhow. The relatively high number of pictures attributes mostly to the fact that some PDF producing programs use pictures for symbols like list bullets. A random sample of 236 captions showed that 15% of the found captions were just random text pieces, like page numbers or single sentences, mostly due to the said symbol pictures. 6% were wrong text that means whole paragraphs of text, just not belonging to the figure. The main reasons here were again symbol pictures, which naturally had no genuine caption and also some cases of figure captions written left or right of the picture. We had 3 cases of duplication, where one figure was internally composed of several pictures, all of which rightly claimed the same caption. We had text conversion problems with only 3 out of these 236 captions. In one no spaces were found, in the second one, some spaces were missing and in the third one some symbols like Δ converted into wrong strings. We had only one case, where the end of the caption was not found correctly. We counted 195 genuine figures in the sample, of which 189 had correctly identified captions. We are still working on a way to sort out which of the images belong to a genuine figure-caption pair and which do not. For a summary confer table 1.

Table 1. Results of Evaluation

No. of paper	No. of papers containing pictures		
188	170 (90%)		
No. of pictures	No. of extractable pictures		
1416	830 (59%)		
No. of captions in sample	short text pieces	wrong text	wrong conversion
236	37 (15%)	17 (7%)	3 (1%)
No. of genuine figures in sample	No. of correctly identified captions to those figures		
195	189 (97%)		

To search for DNAse I footprints, we used the keywords "footprint", "footprinting" and "DNAse". Overall, 184 hits were scored of which 163 actually showed experimental data. As a byproduct, the thumbnails mostly sufficed to make a fast quality assessment. Another positive effect was that the data was much faster available than with the usual method of opening each PDF independently.

The search for EMSAs was a little bit more difficult, since there exist a wide range of naming possiblities. The most significant terms in those names were "shift", "mobility", "EMSA" and "EMS" to catch "EMS assay". We had 91 hits of which 81 were genuine.

Recall could not be tested thoroughly, due the sheer numbers of pictures and the limited time of experts, but the random sample did not include pictures that would not have been found by the keywords, which suggests a rather high recall.

We are still in an early test phase with the user acceptance. For legal reasons we cannot just put the information on the Web and see what is coming, but instead, we only have our local biologist work group as users, who supply us with the literature anyway.

8   Conclusion and Future Work

Although we have just started to explore the possibilities of layout-enhanced analysis of PDF files, our first application looks promising. To bypass the legal problems posed by the copyrights, we plan on publicising a demo version, that does not link to the full text, but to the PubMed entry instead. We also plan to cross-check whether or not the full texts are available on the Internet and then give appropriate addresses, so users can download from the source. This demo version should then be able to give some data about user behaviour.

We are in process of finding more areas of application for our search engine, as we broaden our spectrum of functionalities, especially those mentioned in the sections above, like finding the context a certain figure is mentioned in (eg. "...as you can see in Fig. 2...") to add more text to be searched through and be presented to the user and the extraction of more pictures.

The groundwork of knowing the layout of the publication can also be used for other purposes. On long term, we are working on reading order recognition to improve shallow parsing, which is still a problem in text mining applications [17]. Also, we are investigating the feasibility of a "table search engine" similar to what has already been investigated by [18] for HTML web pages. The overall goal is to make PDF a multifunctional format that can easily be used with any kind of text mining application, just as easily as HTML or plain text.

References

1. PubMed: http://www.ncbi.nlm.nih.gov/pubmed/ (2004)
2. Münch, R., Hiller, K., Barg, H., Heldt, H., Linz, S., Wingender, E., Jahn, D.: Prodoric: prokaryotic database of gene regulation. Nucleic Acids Research **31**(1) (2003) 266–269
3. Faulstich, L.C., Stadler, P.F., Thurner, C., Witwer, C.: litsift: Automated text categorization in bibliographic search. In: Data Mining and Text Mining for Bioinformatics, Workshop at the ECML / PKDD 2003. (2003)
4. Yeh, A., Hirschman, L., Morgan, A.: Evaluation of text data mining for database curation: lessons learned from the kdd challenge cup. Bioinformatics **19**(1) (2003)
5. Shah, P., Perez-Iratxeta, C., Bork, P., Andrade, M.: Information extraction from full text scientific articles: Where are the keywords? BMC Bioinformatics (2003)

6. Adobe Network Solutions: PDF Reference Fourth Edition. http://partners.adobe.com/asn/acrobat/sdk/publicdocs/PDFReference15_v6.pdf (2004)
7. BCL: BCL Jade. http://www.bcltechnologies.com/document/products/jade/jade.htm (2004)
8. Kovacevic, M., Diligenti, M., Gori, M., Milutinovic, V.: Visual Adjacency Multigraphs - a Novel Approach to Web Page Classification. In: Proceedings of SAWM04 workshop, ECML2004. (2004)
9. Litchfield, B.: PDFBox. http://www.pdfbox.org/ or http://sourceforge.net/ (2004)
10. The Apache Software Foundation: Digester. http://jakarta.apache.org/commons/digester/ (2005)
11. Hatcher, E., Gospodnetic, O.: Lucene in Action. Manning Publications (2004)
12. The Apache Software Foundation: Tomcat. http://jakarta.apache.org/tomcat/ (2005)
13. Coward, D., Yoshida, Y.: Java Servlet Specification. http://jcp.org/aboutJava/community-process/final/jsr154/index.html (2003)
14. Deutsch, L.: Deflate compressed data format specification. Request for Comments No 1951, Network Working Group (1996)
15. International Organization for Standardization: ISO/IEC 10918-1:1994: Information technology — Digital compression and coding of continuous-tone still images: Requirements and guidelines. International Organization for Standardization, Geneva, Switzerland (1994)
16. Galperin, M.Y.: The Molecular Biology Database Collection: 2005 update. Nucleic Acids Research **33**(Database-Issue) (2005) 5–24
17. Schmeier, S., Hakenberg, J., Kowald, A., Klipp, E., Leser, U.: Text mining for systems biology using statistical learning methods. In: "3. Workshop des Arbeitskreises Knowledge Discovery". (2003)
18. Wang, Y., Phillips, I.T., Haralick, R.M.: Table detection via probability optimization. In: Proceedings of the 5th IAPR Workshop on Analysis Systems (DAS 2002). (2002) 272–283

Headwords and Suffixes in Biomedical Names

Manabu Torii and Hongfang Liu

Department of Biostatistics, Bioinformatics, and Biomathematics,
Georgetown University Medical Center,
Washington, DC 20007, USA

Abstract. Natural Language Processing (NLP) techniques have been used for the task of extracting and mining knowledge from biomedical literature. One of the critical steps of such a task is biomedical named entity tagging (BNER) which usually contains two steps: the first step is the identification of biomedical names in text and the second is the assignment of semantic classes predefined to names identified by the first step. Headwords and suffixes have been used frequently by BNER systems as features for the assignment of semantic classes to names in text. However, there are few studies to evaluate the performance of headwords and suffixes in predicting semantic classes of biomedical terms utilizing knowledge sources in an unsupervised way. We conducted a study to evaluate the performance of headwords and suffixes using names in the Unified Medical Language System (UMLS) where the semantic classes associated with these names were obtained by modifying an existing UMLS semantic group system and incorporating the GENIA ontology. We define headwords and suffixes that are significantly associated with a specific semantic class as semantic suffixes. The performance of semantic assignment using semantic suffixes achieved an F-measure of 86.4% with a precision of 91.6% and a recall of 81.7%. When applying these semantic suffixes obtained using the UMLS to names extracted from the GENIA corpus, the system achieved an F-measure of 73.4% with a precision of 84.2% and a recall of 65.1% where these performance measures could be improved dramatically when limited to names associated with classes that have the corresponding GENIA types.

1 Introduction

Given the rich amount of biomedical information that resides in biological literature, natural language processing (NLP) techniques are necessary for the task of extracting and mining knowledge from this textual information source [1-3]. One critical step of such a task is biomedical named entity tagging (BNER) [2, 4] which usually consists of two subtasks: i) the identification of biomedical names in text and ii) the assignment of a list of predefined semantic classes to those names. People have investigated these two subtasks either as a whole or individually. For example, in the PASTA system [5], potential name components identified in text using morphological and lexical clues were combined into names and assigned with 12 classes such as proteins, species, atoms, compounds, etc. using a rule-based terminology parser. Lee et al. [6] applied machine learning approaches for BNER and used a different set of

E.G. Bremer et al. (Eds.): KDLL 2006, LNBI 3886, pp. 29–41, 2006.
© Springer-Verlag Berlin Heidelberg 2006

features for each subtask. Torii et al. [7] concentrated on the second subtask and examined the performance of various feature sources for the classification of biomedical names. Nenadic et al. [8] used support vector machine together with various feature selections for the assignment of Gene Ontology classes to gene names.

Most biomedical names are composed of two or more words, and their semantic classes are closely related to their headwords. For example, names with headword as *protein* are proteins and names with headword as *disease* are diseases. Additionally, the semantic classes of some names are closely related to suffixes they bear. For example, a word ending with *onema* usually indicates it is an organism name, like, *Chrysonema* or *Spathionema*, or "itis" indicates a disease, such as *Menengitis*.

There have been several studies utilizing headwords and suffixes for the assignment of semantic classes to biomedical terms [6, 7, 9]. The development of these systems usually requires domain experts to manually craft rules to identify semantic classes of names based on their headwords or suffixes, or to annotate large amount of examples to build machine learning models for predicting semantic classes. Therefore, it is often expensive to build semantic class assignment systems even for specialized domains.

In this paper, we introduce an unsupervised approach to build semantic class assignment systems by exploiting headword and suffix information. We utilized existing online resources in the biomedical domain, and developed semantic class assignment systems that cover the general biomedical domain. Specifically, we used resources available in the Unified Medical Language System (UMLS) [10] and extracted headwords and suffixes that are significantly associated with a specific semantic class, defined them as semantic suffixes. The performance of semantic suffixes was evaluated using reserved test data in the UMLS as well as the GENIA corpus. In the following, we first describe online resources and related work. We then present our methods and results.

2   Online Resources and Related Work

One of the resources used in the study is the Unified Medical Language System (UMLS) which integrates various vocabularies pertaining to biomedicine [10]. The Metathesaurus is one component of the UMLS. It contains information about biomedical concepts and terms from many controlled biomedical vocabularies. The SPECIALIST Lexicon, an English language lexicon, is another component of the UMLS. The last component of the UMLS is the Semantic Network consisting of 134 semantic categories where each concept in the Metathesaurus has been assigned to one or several semantic categories. The UMLS has been explored for developing NLP systems. For example, Johnson developed a method to automatically construct a semantic lexicon based on the Metathesaurus and the SPECIALIST lexicon [11]. Friedman et al. [12] automatically generated a lexicon from the Metathesaurus for a medical language processing system, MedLEE [13]. McCray et al. [14] aggregated UMLS semantic categories to 15 groups to provide a coarser-grained set of semantic classes. Our study here investigates the use of the UMLS to acquire a system that automatically assigns classes to names based on their headwords and suffixes.

Another resource is the GENIA corpus [15]. The current version of the corpus consists of 2,000 MEDLINE abstracts where biomedical concepts related to cell signaling reactions in human were annotated. Those concepts were also categorized into 36 different semantic types according to the GENIA ontology. The GENIA corpus has been used to develop and evaluate NLP systems using supervised machine learning methods [6, 16, 17]. Also, Torii et al. [18] used the GENIA corpus as well as a large set of un-annotated Medline abstracts to show that a system using an un-supervised machine learning method helped extract contextual information classifies biomedical terms into different semantic categories.

Headwords and suffixes have already been reported for semantic class assignment in the field of biomedical text processing [6, 7, 9], as well as in the generic natural language processing field [19, 20]. For example, Narayanaswamy et al. [9] developed a system that identifies biological named entities belonging to five different categories. Identification of categories, as well as extraction of entities from text, relies on manually developed set of rules based on selected words and affixes. They also considered a nearby word of a name for identification of its semantic category. Lee et al. [6], on the other hand, applied a supervised machine learning approach to develop a biological named entity tagging system using Support Vector Machine, and they evaluated their system on the GENIA corpus. They divided the tagging task into two phases: detection of names in text and assignment of semantic categories to detected names. The latter phase was considered as a classification task of detected names. In their classification model using SVM, they used features to indicate if a name contains a certain headword and/or suffix, which are selected based on their frequency in the training corpus. Torii et al. [7] used the GENIA corpus to develop a system that automatically classifies biomedical terms into different semantic categories. In their work, they merged subtypes of protein type, DNA type, and RNA type in the GENIA ontology, and used 22 semantic types. Their system exploited headwords and suffixes of terms, nearby words, as well as several heuristics to predict semantic categories of terms, and it achieved an F-measure of 86% in 10-fold cross validation test.

Our study is different from related studies since we focused on extracting semantic suffixes in an unsupervised manner using the UMLS and evaluated the prediction power of these semantic suffixes. Since the UMLS is a comprehensive resource in the general biomedical domain, the methods can be applied generally to assign semantic classes to biomedical names.

3 Methods

Our study involves several steps. We first built up a list of semantic classes by modifying the UMLS semantic group system proposed by McCray [14] and incorporating GENIA ontology. In McCray's work, genes are in a class called Genes and Molecular sequences while gene products are in a class called Chemicals and Drugs. However, since genes and gene products are usually named after each other and most BNER systems do not distinguish them, we modified the UMLS semantic group system so that genes and gene products are in the same class. Secondly, we normalized names by grouping textual variants and removing short endings (e.g., *1*, *A* or *II*). There are two reasons. First, our study was to identify headwords and suffixes associated with semantic classes while most of these short endings do not indicate semantic classes. Secondly, most BNER systems can handle textual variants, and grouping textual variants allows us to obtain more meaningful statistics. The third step was to derive semantic class assignment systems based on the co-occurrence information between headwords/suffixes and semantic classes. The last step includes the evaluation of these systems using reserved test data in the UMLS as well as the GENIA corpus.

To avoid using the same data for training and testing, names in the Metathesaurus were split into two portions, UMLS_train and UMLS_test. Also, type-annotated names extracted from the GENIA corpus were split into two portions, GENIA_train and GENIA_test. GENIA_train was used for the determination of mapping between GENIA types and the UMLS semantic categories. The obtained mapping scheme was applied to GENIA_test, and the resulting corpus was used for the evaluation of the class assignment systems trained using UMLS_train.

3.1 Obtaining a List of Semantic Classes

Based on the definitions of semantic categories provided in the UMLS Semantic Network (SRDEF), we modified McCray's semantic group system by moving gene products related UMLS semantic categories (e.g., Enzyme (T126)) to the class Genes and Molecular Sequences and renamed it as Genes and Gene Products. Such modified semantic groups were used as the list of semantic classes in the study.

Note that the GENIA ontology and the UMLS Semantic Network are in different granularities. Sometimes, GENIA ontology has finer granularity than the UMLS. For example, the UMLS semantic category Cell (T025) contains concepts from two GENIA categories (i.e., cell_line and cell_type). Sometimes, the UMLS has finer granularity. For example, "Other_names" category in the GENIA contains names of diseases (e.g., Disease or Syndrome (T047)) as well as procedure names (e.g., Laboratory Procedure (T059)). Based on the above observation, we need a method to map GENIA ontology into the list of semantic classes obtained.

The mapping of GENIA types onto the modified UMLS semantic categories was obtained using the co-occurrence statistics of common names in the UMLS and GENIA_train. For example, the string *lipoxygenase* is associated with two categories in GENIA, protein_family_or_group and protein_molecule and one modified UMLS semantic category (i.e., Genes and Gene Products). Then the co-occurrence of protein_family_or_group and Genes and Gene Products and the co-occurrence of protein_molecule and Genes and Gene Products would be increased by 1. Based on the co-occurrence information obtained, we mapped each GENIA type to the significant majority semantic class. For GENIA types that do not have the significant majority semantic class (e.g., Other_names), we ignored them in our mapping.

3.2 Filtering and Normalizing Names

We used the following process to obtain a collection of names from the Metathesaurus that we used to extract headwords and suffixes. Since headwords in names containing commas and hyphens are not easy to detect, we first filtered out names that contain commas and hyphens (except names where hyphen connects two words with no space in between, e.g, *Bassen-Kornzweig syndrome*). Additionally, names containing prepositions, conjunctions, or certain other pre-selected words such as *which*, *that*, and *how* etc. were also filtered out for the same reason. Next, we normalized the remaining terms using the following normalization procedure: i) changing all names into lower case, ii) normalizing syntactic variants using the Specialist Lexicon, iii) unifying punctuation marks, and iv) removing short endings and GREEK alphabets. Note that most of these short endings are single alphabet letters (e.g., *A*, *C*), or Roman Numerals (e.g., *II*, *IV*), or abbreviations. For example, *Bassen-Kornzweig Syndrome BASSEN KORNZWEIG SYNDROME*, *Bassen Kornzweig syndrome*, and *Bassen Kornzweig Syndrome* are unified as *bassen kornzweig syndrome* while *death receptor 3*, *death receptor 4*, and *death receptor 5* were normalized as *death receptor*. Finally, we filtered out names where headwords of them (the rightmost words after normalization) were less than four-letter long, or were originally all upper-case letters (i.e., acronyms). Denote the resulting collection of normalized names as NNAMES. The same normalization procedure was also applied to names extracted from the GENIA corpus.

The above process is necessary for acquiring a collection of headwords easily and accurately (i.e., considering words at the right end of names as headwords). It also removes undesirable redundancies in the collection. For example, *Chromosome 1*, *Chromosome 2*, *Chromosome 3*, ..., are normalized to a single entry *Chromosome*.

3.3 Obtaining Semantic Suffixes

As we have mentioned, semantic classes of biomedical terms are often related to their headwords. For example, names with the headword "inhibitor" (e.g., *Acetylcholinesterase Inhibitors or alpha 1-Protease Inhibitor*) are mostly assigned with the category Pharmacologic Substance (T121) and/or Amino Acid, Peptide, or Protein (T116) in the UMLS and such names are assigned with the type other_organic_compound in the GENIA corpus. In some cases, the headword alone is not sufficient to determine the semantic classes of the named entities. For instance, phrases ending with the words *cell clone* and *DNA clone* often belong to different semantic categories in the domain. Besides headwords, sometimes semantic categories of names can be inferred from their suffixes of headwords. For instance, names with the headword ending with "-octye" (e.g., *Acanthocyte*) are assigned with the type Cell (T025) in the UMLS, and such names are assigned with cell_type or cell_line in the GENIA corpus. Note that the suffix "-cyte" derived from the Greek word "kytos" is known to denote a cell. We considered the rightmost words of the normalized names as the headwords. Therefore, these headwords can also be treated as suffixes. We needed to derive a list of headwords and suffixes that significantly associate with specific semantic classes. Denote such headwords and suffixes as semantic suffixes.

In order to obtain semantic suffixes, we used NNAMES. Generally, the semantic category of each normalized name could be easily derived by using the mapping scheme obtained in Section 3.2. However, some special treatments were needed as indicating in the following:

- Ignoring non-leaf UMLS semantic categories - The UMLS Semantic Network is a directed acyclic digraph while descendent leaf nodes of the same semantic category may be mapped onto multiple modified UMLS semantic groups in our mapping scheme based on McCray's work. For example, the non-leaf UMLS semantic category Organic Chemical (T109) is mapped onto the semantic group Chemical & Drugs (CHEM), while its two descendent leaf nodes Amino Acid, Peptide, or Protein (T116) and Carbohydrate (T118) are mapped onto Genes and Gene Products (GP) and CHEM, respectively. Such a mapping introduces undesirable ambiguity. For instance, in Metathesaurus, the term *glomecidin* is annotated with the two categories T109 and T116, which are mapped onto CHEM and GP, and hence the term is considered to be ambiguous. In this case, however, T116 should override its ancestor type T109, and the term can be assigned only with GP. Moreover, given terms annotated with T109 and T116 (e.g., *glomecidin*) as well as a fair number of terms annotated with T109 and T118 (e.g., *gleptoferron*) in the Metathesaurus, we notice the notion of T109 should span those of T116 and T118 both, which prohibits T109 to be mapped only to CHEM. To avoid this problem, we did not use non-leaf UMLS semantic categories (e.g., T109).

- Chemical Viewed Functionally v.s. Chemical Viewed Structurally - We noticed that many chemical concepts are assigned with two UMLS semantic categories belonging to the category Chemical Viewed Functionally (T120) and Chemical Viewed Structurally (T104), respectively. In our mapping scheme, the categories belonging to the former are mapped onto CHEM and those belonging to the latter are mapped onto GP. Since names assigned with these two UMLS categories are mostly assigned with GENIA types that are related to genes and gene products, we assigned GP if a name was assigned with two categories belonging to these chemical super categories.

- Ambiguous Terms - Some terms in the UMLS have multiple senses. The disambiguation task depends on the effective use of contextual information of terms. For names associated with multiple senses, if those senses ended up with the same semantic class, we kept them. Otherwise, we ignored those terms. Though ambiguous terms play a crucial role in biological text mining, we note that the proportion of ambiguous terms in the Metathesaurus is very small, 0.6%, as in Section 4.

We then obtained a collection of names where each name was associated with a specific semantic class. In order to determine semantic suffixes from these names, we stored these names in a TRIE structure. Since words in a name that are closely associated with its semantic class are usually at most two words from the right end of the name, the building process stops when reaching the rightmost two words of a name. An example of TRIE structure (http://en.wikipedia.org/wiki/Trie) is shown in Figure 1. Each node of the structure is associated with a certain suffix, say *-ase*, and its children indicate the variation of letters that could precede the suffix, say *e*, *g*, and *n*, which may be derived from the stored names such as *amyloid disease*, *ligase*, *dehydrogenase* or *monooxygenase*. Each node stores the number of times the associated suffix is observed among the names stored in the structure, and the node also stores how many names are assigned with a certain semantic class among all the names having the associated suffix. Therefore, at each node, we can evaluate one suffix string associated with the node. We can calculate how often each semantic class is associated with the suffix, i.e., P(*class*|*suffix*). If this likelihood value is above a certain threshold, we record the suffix as an indicator of the corresponding semantic class (i.e., a semantic suffix). Let us call this threshold the accuracy threshold. Besides the accuracy threshold, we also defined the threshold on the frequency of suffixes, i.e., we do not consider a suffix as a semantic suffix unless it appears in names frequently as specified by this threshold. Let us call this threshold as the frequency threshold.

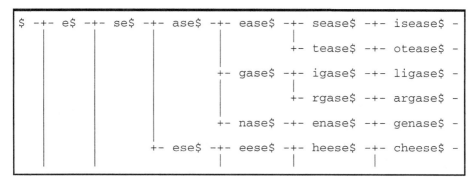

Fig. 1. TRIE structure: Each node in the structure is associated with a unique suffix of names stored in the structure. The symbol $ indicates the end of a suffix string.

After obtaining semantic suffixes, the use of semantic suffixes for class assignment is straightforward. Given a name with an unknown semantic class, we first normalize the name, and then look up the longest semantic suffix of the name. If such a semantic suffix is found, we assign the semantic class associated with the semantic suffix to the name. If no such semantic suffix is found, we consider its semantic class cannot be determined using the semantic suffixes learned.

3.4 Evaluation

In order to evaluate our method, we obtained a list of biomedical names, NNAMES, derived from the UMLS Metathesaurus, each of which was associated with predefined semantic categories (see Section 3.2). We randomly chose 10,000 normalized names from NNAMES, and reserved them as test data (UMLS_test). To the remaining names in NNAMES (UMLS_train), we applied our semantic suffix extraction process (see Section 3.3), and recorded the results. Then, we evaluated the category assignment system that utilizes the extracted semantic suffixes over UMLS_test. For instance, the suffix extraction process recognized the sequence *amoeba* as a semantic suffix associated with the category Living Being (LIVB), which was witnessed by the fact that 38 names in UMLS_train have the suffix/headword *amoeba* in their rightmost words and are all assigned with the semantic category LIVB, e.g., *Platyamoeba*, *Rhizamoeba*, *Leptomyxid amoeba*, etc. In testing, two names in UMLS_test that have the suffix *amoeba* in their rightmost words were detected. To these names, the category assignment system assigned LIVB according to the association between the suffix and the category learned from UMLS_train. To test the effect of different threshold settings, we tested different combinations of accuracy threshold values and frequency threshold values.

We also evaluated the class assignment system over GENIA_test, the list of normalized names annotated with GENIA types that were extracted from 1,500 Medline abstracts in the GENIA corpus. According to the mapping table between GENIA types and UMLS semantic categories, which was obtained by using GENIA_train (see Section 3.1), we replaced types assigned to names in GENIA_test with the corresponding semantic classes, and evaluated the performance of the class assignment system just as before.

4 Results and Discussion

Table 1 shows the list of semantic classes as well as the ratio of names in GENIA_train that could be mapped to the corresponding significant majority semantic classes. The first and second columns show the information about these semantic classes. The third column indicates the corresponding UMLS semantic categories (denoted using regular expression) and the last column shows the mapping information of the GENIA types to the semantic classes. The ratio following the GENIA type indicates how well it mapped. For example, there are 27 Body_part terms in GENIA that could be mapped to the UMLS where 25 of them fall into the ANAT category. Note that Other_name GENIA type could not be mapped to one specific UMLS semantic group.

We obtained 431,699 different normalized name strings from the Metathesaurus, each of which was associated with semantic classes. Of these name entries, 2,721 name strings (0.6%) were associated with more than one semantic class (ambiguous names). We did not use these ambiguous names in our experiment. Similarly, of 10,000 normalized UMLS name strings reserved for testing purpose, 78 names are associated with more than one class, and hence the actual evaluation were conducted on 9,922 name strings. Table 2 shows the performance of suffix-based category assignment systems with different combinations of the accuracy threshold (0.75, 0.85, 0.90 and 0.95) and the frequency threshold (1, 5, and 10) when evaluating on UMLS_test. Table 3 shows assignment results on each category, where the accuracy threshold is 0.80 and the frequency threshold is 1.

We extracted 27,448 different names from GENIA_test. We ignored names associated with GENIA type Other_name, and obtained a total of 10,651 different name strings after normalization. The performance of category assignment systems based on semantic suffixes extracted from UMLS_train is shown in Table 4. Table 5 shows the performance of the assignment systems on each semantic category on GENIA_test.

Note that our results on the GENIA corpus are not comparable to existing BNER studies using the GENIA corpus (e.g., [6, 21]) since our focus here is strictly on the classification task (i.e., the second subtask). Additionally, semantic classes considered in this study are much broader than those in related work.

Table 2 shows that semantic classes of biomedical names could be predicted with high precisions and high recalls based on their headwords and suffixes. However, Table 3 implies that it is difficult to achieve high recalls on some rare classes such as ACTI (Activities and Behaviors), GEOG (Geographic Areas), ORGA (Organizations), and PHEN (Phenomena). The reasons for these low recalls are due to unique names for a few classes, e.g., *North Carolina* [GEOG]. But there are some other causes. For instance, given the name *Histoplasmosis test positive* [PHEN], the suffix extraction process falsely recognized *positive* as its headword. Even if the system could recognize *test* as its headword, *test* should not be closely associated with PHEN in general. In fact, this could be the reason why it is difficult to achieve high recalls for the classes CONC (Concepts and Ideas), e.g., *Attitude changed* [CONC] where *changed* is not the headword, and even the true headword *attitude* is often associated with PHYS rather than CONC in the training data.

Table 1. Modified UMLS semantic groups and the mapping of the UMLS semantic categories and GENIA types

Type	Definition	UMLS	GENIA
ACTI	Activities & Behavior	T05[1-7] T06[46]	
ANAT	Anatomy	T01[8] T02[2-6,9] T031	Body_part (25/27) Cell_* (123/131) Tissue (23/26)
CHEM	Chemicals & Drugs	T11[1,5,8] T12[2-4,7] T13[0,1] T19[5-7] T200	Inorganic (10/11) Atom (12/12) Other_organic_compound (50/83)
CONC	Concepts & Ideas	T0[77-82] T089 T102 T[169-171] T185	
DEVI	Devices	T07[45]	
DISO	Disorders	T0[19-20] T03[37] T0[46-50] T184 T19[01]	
GEOG	Georgraphic Areas	T083	
GP	Genes&Gene Products	T028 T08[6,7] T11[0,4,6] T12[5,6,9] T192	Amino_acid_monomer (14/14) DNA_* (167/184) Lipid (18/21) Nucleotide (10/10) Peptide (15/17) Polynucleotide (6/7) Protein_* (694/716) RNA_* (3/3)
LIVB	Living Beings	T00[4,5,7,9] T01[3,6] T09[7-9] T10[0-1]	Mono_cell (9/10) Multi_cell (19/24) Virus (19/24)
OBJC	Objects	T07[1-3] T16[78]	
OCCU	Occupations	T09[01]	
ORGA	Organizations	T09[2-5]	
PHEN	Phenomena	T034 T038 T0[67-70]	
PHYS	Physiology	T04[0-5] T201	
PROC	Procedures	T0[58-63] T065	

Table 2. The overall performance of suffix-based category assignment systems using various combinations of accuracy thresholds (AT) and frequency thresholds (FT) where P stands for precision, R stands for recall, and F stands for F-Measure

FT	1			5			10		
AT	P	R	F	P	R	F	P	R	F
0.75	90.3	**82.0**	86.0	91.3	79.9	85.3	91.7	76.6	83.5
0.80	91.6	81.7	**86.4**	92.7	79.0	85.3	92.9	74.9	83.0
0.85	92.5	80.8	86.2	94.3	76.2	84.3	94.4	72.8	82.2
0.90	93.4	79.5	85.9	95.6	73.7	83.2	95.7	70.1	80.9
0.95	95.1	77.2	85.3	96.7	69.4	80.8	**97.0**	64.3	77.3

Table 3. The performance of semantic suffixes on UMLS_test with respect to each specific semantic group where the accuracy threshold is 0.8 and frequency threshold is 1

Type	Total	Precision	Recall	F-Measure
ACTI	56	55.9	33.9	42.2
ANAT	810	90.5	80.0	84.9
CHEM	1812	91.0	81.0	85.7
CONC	148	82.1	43.2	56.6
DEVI	6	100	100	100
DISO	814	89.1	82.4	85.6
GEOG	28	85.7	21.4	34.3
GP	1909	92.4	80.1	85.8
LIVB	2897	94.9	88.8	91.8
OBJC	60	88.0	36.7	51.8
OCCU	12	83.3	83.3	83.3
ORGA	24	86.7	54.2	66.7
PHEN	52	84.6	42.3	56.4
PHYS	437	87.2	78.0	82.4
PROC	857	88.7	83.0	85.7
Total	9922	91.6	81.7	86.4

Note that sometimes, the semantic class of a name cannot be detected by its headwords and suffixes. For example, given the name *Severe multi tissue damage lower arm*, the semantic group Disorders (DISO) may be implied by the word *damage* rather than the headword *arm*. These names prevent the extraction of *arm* as a semantic suffix for ANAT, which is the right category of, for example, *Right upper arm*.

Table 4. The performance of semantic suffixes when training using the Metathesaurus and testing using GENIA names

FT	1			5			10		
AT	P	R	F	P	R	F	P	R	F
0.75	79.7	65.4	71.8	84.9	65.6	**74.0**	84.2	60.4	70.4
0.80	80.7	**66.3**	72.7	87.1	63.1	73.2	87.5	57.5	69.4
0.85	82.2	65.9	73.2	88.2	59.1	70.8	90.6	55.0	68.4
0.90	84.0	63.0	72.0	90.8	47.7	62.5	91.0	43.1	58.5
0.95	83.5	51.7	63.9	91.0	41.6	57.1	**91.1**	35.5	51.1

Table 5. The performance of semantic suffixes on GENIA_test with respect to each specific semantic group where the accuracy threshold is 0.75 and frequency threshold is 5

Type	Total	Precision	Recall	F-Measure
ANAT	2849	88.4	73.9	80.5
CHEM	777	45.1	24.7	31.9
GP	6420	93.9	68.8	79.5
LIVB	605	63.0	45.3	52.7
Total	10651	84.2	65.1	73.4

The precision and the recall of semantic suffixes were lower for names extracted from GENIA_test, compared to those for names in UMLS_test. There are several reasons. One could be ascribed to the specialized domain of the GENIA corpus. Since the GENIA abstracts were collected using specific keywords (i.e., *Human, blood cells,* and *Transcription Factor*), terms used in the abstracts as well as semantic groups were specialized in a certain domain. For instance, in the GENIA corpus, terms with the headword *member* usually refer to a member of a certain protein family, e.g., *NF-kappaB/Rel family members.* Hence, they are assigned as GP (i.e., Genes and Gene products). On the other hand, in the UMLS, terms with the headword *member(s)* could be associated with Professional or Occupational Group (T097), Population Group (T098), Family Group (T099), and several other categories including Amino Acid, Peptide, or Protein (T116). Due to the wide coverage of the UMLS, some semantic suffixes in GENIA (e.g., *region, site,* and *domain*) cannot be detected as semantic suffixes using the UMLS. To test how well semantic suffixes performed when limited to a specific domain, we applied the extraction program on names in UMLS_train that associated with four semantic classes (ANAT, CHEM, GP, and LIVB) and then tested using names in GENIA_test with three frequency thresholds (1, 5, and 10) and one accuracy threshold (0.95), the F-measure increased from 63.9% to 77.2%, 57.1% to 71.3%, and 51.1% to 64.2% respectively.

5 Conclusion and Future Work

We have presented here a study about the prediction power of headwords and suffixes for the assignment of semantic classes in biomedical names. A list of semantic classes covering the general biomedical domain was derived using online resources. Headwords and suffixes significantly associated with a specific semantic class were obtained and semantic class assignment systems were then built for the general biomedical domain. From the study, we found that headwords and suffixes can be used to build semantic class assignment systems and achieve reasonable performance. The study indicates that the prediction power of semantic suffixes increases when limited to a specific domain. Furthermore, our suffix extraction method currently does not take the number of occurrence information of names in a corpus into consideration. Future work would be to extract semantic suffixes by taking such occurrence information in a corpus into account.

Acknowledgement. The study was supported by IIS-0430743 from the National Science Foundation.

References

1. Hirschman L, Park JC, Tsujii J, Wong L, Wu CH: **Accomplishments and challenges in literature data mining for biology.** *Bioinformatics* 2002, **18**(12):1553-1561.
2. Hirschman L, Yeh A, Blaschke C, Valencia A: **Overview of BioCreAtIvE: critical assessment of information extraction for biology.** *BMC Bioinformatics* 2005, **6 Suppl 1**:S1.
3. Shatkay H, Feldman R: **Mining the biomedical literature in the genomic era: an overview.** *J Comput Biol* 2003, **10**(6):821-855.
4. Krauthammer M, Nenadic G: **Term identification in the biomedical literature.** *J Biomed Inform* 2004, **37**(6):512-526.
5. Gaizauskas R, Demetriou G, Artymiuk PJ, Willett P: **Protein structures and information extraction from biological texts: the PASTA system.** *Bioinformatics* 2003, **19**(1):135-143.
6. Lee KJ, Hwang YS, Kim S, Rim HC: **Biomedical named entity recognition using two-phase model based on SVMs.** *J Biomed Inform* 2004, **37**(6):436-447.
7. Torii M, Kamboj S, Vijay-Shanker K: **Using name-internal and contextual features to classify biological terms.** *J Biomed Inform* 2004, **37**(6):498-511.
8. Nenadic G, Spasic I, Ananiadou S: **Terminology-driven mining of biomedical literature.** *Bioinformatics* 2003, **19**(8):938-943.
9. Narayanaswamy M, Ravikumar KE, Vijay-Shanker K: **A biological named entity recognizer.** *Pac Symp Biocomput* 2003:427-438.
10. Bodenreider O: **The Unified Medical Language System (UMLS): integrating biomedical terminology.** *Nucleic Acids Res* 2004, **32 Database issue**:D267-270.
11. Johnson SB: **A semantic lexicon for medical language processing.** *J Am Med Inform Assoc* 1999, **6**(3):205-218.
12. Friedman C, Liu H, Shagina L, Johnson S, Hripcsak G: **Evaluating the UMLS as a source of lexical knowledge for medical language processing.** *Proc AMIA Symp* 2001:189-193.
13. Friedman C, Alderson PO, Austin JH, Cimino JJ, Johnson SB: **A general natural-language text processor for clinical radiology.** *J Am Med Inform Assoc* 1994, **1**(2):161-174.

14. McCray AT, Burgun A, Bodenreider O: **Aggregating UMLS semantic types for reducing conceptual complexity**. *Medinfo* 2001, **10**(Pt 1):216-220.
15. Kim JD, Ohta T, Tateisi Y, Tsujii J: **GENIA corpus--semantically annotated corpus for bio-textmining**. *Bioinformatics* 2003, **19 Suppl 1**:i180-182.
16. Zhou G, Zhang J, Su J, Shen D, Tan C: **Recognizing names in biomedical texts: a machine learning approach**. *Bioinformatics* 2004, **20**(7):1178-1190.
17. Tsuruoka Y, Tsujii J: **Improving the performance of dictionary-based approaches in protein name recognition**. *J Biomed Inform* 2004, **37**(6):461-470.
18. Torii M, Vijay-Shanker K: **Using Unlabeled MEDLINE Abstracts for Biological Named Entity Classification**. In: *Proceedings of Genome Informatics Workshop: 2002*; 2002: 567-568.
19. Cucerzan S, Yarowsky D: **Language Independent Named Entity Recognition Combining Morphological and Contextual Evidence**. In: *Proceedings of the Workshop on Very Large Cor- pora at the Conference on Empirical Methods in NLP: 1999*; 1999.
20. Collins M, Singer Y: **Unsupervised models for named entity classification**. In: *Empirical Methods in Natural Language Processing and Very Large Corpora: 1999*; 1999.
21. Kazama J, Makino T, Ohta Y, Tsujii J: **Tuning support vector machine for biomedical named entity recognition**. In: *Workshop on Natural Language Processing in the Biomedical Domain, ACL: 2002*; 2002.

A Tree Kernel-Based Method
for Protein-Protein Interaction Mining
from Biomedical Literature

Jae-Hong Eom, Sun Kim, Seong-Hwan Kim, and Byoung-Tak Zhang

Biointelligence Laboratory,
School of Computer Science and Engineering,
Seoul National University, Seoul 151-744, South Korea
{jheom, skim, shkim, btzhang}@bi.snu.ac.kr

Abstract. As genomic research advances, the knowledge discovery from
a large collection of scientific papers becomes more important for efficient
biological and biomedical research. Even though current databases continue to update new protein-protein interactions, valuable information
still remains in biomedical literature. Thus data mining techniques are
required to extract the information. In this paper, we present a tree
kernel-based method to mine protein-protein interactions from biomedical literature. The tree kernel is designed to consider grammatical structures for given sentences. A support vector machine classifier is combined
with the tree kernel and trained on predefined interaction corpus and set
of interaction patterns. Experimental results show that the proposed
method gives promising results by utilizing the structure patterns.

1 Introduction

Since protein-protein interactions play key roles in various biological processes
[1], detail analysis of these interactions would significantly contribute to the
understanding of the biological phenomena. As genomic research advances, the
knowledge discovery from a large collection of scientific papers becomes more
important to support biological and biomedical research. Thus, how to extract
protein interactions from biomedical literature has been an active research subject over recent years.

There are many accomplishments in literature data mining for biological data
analysis and in most cases they focus on protein interaction extraction. But, the
protein interaction data is still accumulated manually in biological databases.
Furthermore, scientists sometime continue to publish their discoveries on new
protein interactions and modifying previous results in scientific papers without
submitting to the public databases [2]. Therefore, a lot of interaction data still
exist only in text materials.

Protein interaction extraction systems widely adopt natural language processing (NLP) techniques. The NLP approaches can be regarded as parsing-based
methods and both full and shallow parsing strategies have been performed in

E.G. Bremer et al. (Eds.): KDLL 2006, LNBI 3886, pp. 42–52, 2006.

previous studies. Yakushiji et al. [3] used a general full parser with grammars for biomedical domain to extract interaction events by filling sentences into augmented structures. Park et al. [4] proposed bidirectional incremental full parsing with combinatory categorical grammar (CCG) which localizes target verbs and then scans the left and right neighborhood of the verb respectively to find interaction events in the sentences. Temkin et al. [5] also utilized a lexical analyzer and context-free grammar (CFG) to extract gene, protein, and small molecule interactions with recall rate of 63.9% and precision rate of 70.2%. Similarly, preposition-based parsing to generate templates also proposed by Leroy et al. [6] and they achieved precision of 70% for biomedical literature abstract processing. For a partial parsing method, Pustejovsky et al. [7] used the relational parsing for the inhibition relation with recall rate of 57%. But, these methods are inherently complicated, requiring many resources, and the performance is not satisfactory as yet.

In this paper, we extract protein-protein interactions from biomedical literature using a tree kernel-based method, which utilizes grammatical structure of sentences directly. A support vector machine (SVM) with the tree kernel is used to discriminate interaction and non-interaction data from predefined interaction corpus and set of interaction patterns. The proposed approach exploits part-of-speech (POS) tags and text structures to improve extraction performance.

Here, we address how the tree kernel can be used to extract protein interactions and how to the extraction performance can be further improved. This paper is organized as follows. In Section 2, the basic concept of kernel method and its types are described. The tree kernel for protein-protein interaction extraction is explained in Section 3. In Section 4, we show the experimental results of protein interaction extraction. Finally, in Section 5, we present concluding remarks and draw future directions.

2   Kernel Method

An object can be transformed into a collection of features $f_1, \ldots, f_N$, which produce N-dimensional feature vectors. However, it is difficult to express data via features. For example, feature-based representations in NLP problems produce inherently local representations of objects and it is computationally infeasible to generate features involving long-range dependencies.

Kernel methods are an attractive alternative of feature-based approaches. Kernel methods retain the original representation of objects and use the object in algorithms only via computing a kernel function between a pair of objects. A kernel function is a similarity function which has certain properties. That is, kernel function K over the object space X is binary function $K : X \times X \rightarrow [0, \infty]$ mapping a pair of objects $x, y \in X$ to their similarity score $K(x, y)$. This is embedding procedure of data items (e.g. genes, proteins, molecular compounds, etc.) into a vector space F, called feature space, and searching for linear relation in the feature space. This embedding is defined implicitly, by specifying an inner product for the feature space via a symmetric and positive semidefinite kernel function: $K(x, y) = \langle \Phi(x), \Phi(y) \rangle$, where $\Phi(x)$ and $\Phi(y)$ are the embeddings of data items, x and y [8].

Kernel functions implicitly calculate the inner product of feature vectors in high-dimensional feature spaces by projecting all objects from their original low-dimensional spaces. That is, there exist features $f(\cdot) = (f_1(\cdot), f_2(\cdot), \ldots)$, $f_i : X \to R$, so that $K(x, y) = \langle f(x), f(y) \rangle$. Conversely, given features $f(\cdot) = (f_1(\cdot), f_2(\cdot), \ldots)$, a function defined as a dot product of the corresponding feature vectors is necessarily a kernel function [8].

In many cases, it is possible to compute the dot product of certain features without enumerating all the features. One good example is the subsequence kernels. In the subsequence kernels, the inputs are strings of characters, and the kernel function computes the number of common subsequences between two strings, where each subsequence match is additionally decreased by the factor reflecting how spread out the matched subsequence in the original sequences [9]. Despite of an exponential increase in number of features (subsequences), it is possible to compute kernel matrix in polynomial time. Therefore, one can exploit long-range features without enumerating the features explicitly.

There are a number of learning algorithms that operate only by using the dot product of examples. The models produced by the learning algorithms are also expressed by dot product of examples. Substituting a particular kernel functions in place of dot product defines a specific instantiation of such learning algorithms. The algorithms which process examples only via computing their dot products are sometimes called dual learning algorithms. The SVM [10] is known as the learning method that not only allows for a dual formulation, but also provides a rigorous rationale for resisting over-fitting. For the kernel-based algorithms working in extremely rich feature spaces, it is crucial to deal with the problem of over-fitting problems. Many experimental results indicate that the SVM is able to generalize classification boundary very well and avoid over-fitting in high dimensional feature spaces. Thus, we use the SVM method with the tree kernel to extract protein interactions.

3   Tree Kernel for Protein-Protein Interaction Extraction

3.1   Tree Kernel

There have been many approaches for text classification using kernel methods. The BOW (bag-of-word) kernel, which uses word frequency vectors as features and calculates inner products to get their similarities, is a typical form of kernel classification methods [11].

Kernel-based approaches using simple word distribution of documents cannot make use of the grammatical structure, however, new kernel method which utilizes the structural information have been proposed in Collins [12]. The sequence kernel considers the data as a sequence of characters and the common subsequences as attributes. It calculates kernel value by counting these common subsequences. The kernels which calculate structural similarity in a recursive manner are called 'convolution kernel' [13].

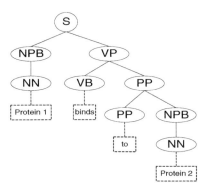

Fig. 1. An example of parsing tree

The tree kernel is a convolution kernel and naturally uses the grammatical structure. The tree kernel represents a structure with a tree form and numbers the child nodes of parent node by its order. A parsing tree represents the text and the structural information. Figure 1 shows the parsing tree of "protein1 binds to protein2." In the tree kernel, kernel value is evaluated by summing up the number of common subtrees between two trees. Consequently, the tree kernel can be used to calculate the structural similarity effectively.

A tree represents as a vector of subtree consisting of corresponding tree itself through high dimensional feature mapping:

$$\Phi(\text{Tree } T) = (subTree(\text{type } 1), \ldots, subTtree(\text{type } n)), \tag{1}$$

where $subTree(\text{type } n)$ is the number of subtree of node type n.

The kernel function is defined as follows:

$$K(T_1, T_2) = \langle \Phi(T_1) \cdot \Phi(T_2) \rangle = \sum_l \Phi(T_1)[i] \times \Phi(T_2)[i] \tag{2}$$

$$= \sum_{n_1 \in N_1} \sum_{n_2 \in N_2} \sum_i I_i(n_1) \times I_i(n_2), \tag{3}$$

where N_1 and N_2 represent the set of all possible nodes of tree T_1 and T_2, and $I_i(n)$ is an indicator function which has 1 if subtree of type i is started from root node n, 0 otherwise.

The number of subtrees with type i in T is calculated by $\Phi(T)[i] = \sum_{n \in N} I_i(n)$. It means that the total number of nodes in tree T which have subtrees with type i. The inner product between two trees, having its features as the all possible sub-trees, is computed by the following recursive way and it is known to be calculated in polynomial time.

1. If the form of the children nodes of n_1 and n_2 are different,

$$NumComSubt(n_1, n_2) = 0 \tag{4}$$

2. If the form of the children nodes of n_1 and n_2 are identical (including their order) and they are leaf nodes (POS tag),

$$NumComSubt(n_1, n_2) = \lambda \tag{5}$$

3. For all other cases,

$$NumComSubt(n_1, n_2) = \prod_j (1 + NumComSubt(ch(n_1)_j, ch(n_2)_j)), \quad (6)$$

where $ch(n_1)_j$ is the j-th child of node n_1, $ch(n_2)_j$ is the j-th child of node n_2, and $NumComSubt(n_1, n_2) = \lambda \sum_i I_i(n_1) \times I_i(n_2)$. The parameter λ, $0 < \lambda \leq 1$, is used to consider the relative importance of tree fragment according to its length and is set to '1' when the size of tree fragments is not considered.

3.2   Applying Tree Kernel

We can improve some degree of extraction performance simply by using a set of patterns or rules because the protein interactions are represented by typical forms in many cases [2][14]. Generally, text sentences are generated from specific rules such as grammar, then they form grammatical structures. Thus we can utilize the structural properties from texts.

In this paper, we use a tree kernel which calculates tree similarity implicitly without explicit rules or templates. By using the tree kernel we can compute the similarity between two parse trees without modifying their structures. On the other hand, it does not necessarily need to analyze full tree to extract protein-protein interactions because the result can be decided by only sub-structure including the interactions. Therefore, we only use the minimum subtrees that have two proteins from full trees. This work helps to improve computational efficiency and accurate extraction.

3.3   Adding Semantic Information by Tag-Transformation

In the parsing tree, the tag information at leaf nodes plays an important role to identify structure patterns, then we can add simple semantic information for protein or interaction by modifying their POS tags. Possible two candidates are 'NN' tag for protein and 'VB' tag for interaction. Firstly, we can modify 'NN' tag of protein to 'PTN' to represent explicitly which is a protein in tree structure level. This tag modification would not have any advantage when the structure of positive sentence (which contains valid protein interaction) and negative sentence (which does not contain any protein interaction) are totally different. But, if both sentences from positive and negative examples have similar structure and the modified POS tags are used, we could discriminate protein interactions more easily.

Secondly, we can modify interaction-related verbs and nouns. A list of interaction verbs representing protein interactions are well studied in many researches. We have chosen interaction-related verbs determined by referencing these resources and by human experts. A POS tag for interaction-related verbs is transformed by adding '-I' (from 'VB' to 'VB-I') to differentiate protein interaction verbs from general verbs. A POS tag for interaction-related nouns is also transformed in the same way, from 'NN' to 'NN-I', to distinguish deverbal nouns (e.g., a noun 'regulation' formed from a verb 'regulate') from other normal nouns. These modified tags are used to give rich information when we calculate kernel value to compare similarity of subtree structures. In the experiments, we examine the impact of using the semantic information.

4   Experimental Results

4.1   Data Set

In order to generate the data set, we have first found the abstracts with the keyword, 'protein interaction' or 'protein-protein interaction' in PubMed. Next, five proteins (TRPC, CREB, ERK, FOS, and EGR) have been selected as queries among proteins that have over 2,000 relevant abstracts. More than 10,000 abstracts were retrieved by the five queries, and segmented into sentences, where the number of sentences was about 100,000. To make the problem more difficult, we discarded any sentence which contains less than two protein names or no interaction-related word. Note that the sentences which contain at least two protein names and one interaction-related word may not include protein-protein interactions at all. Finally, the sentences which include protein-protein interactions were labeled as 'positive', otherwise labeled as 'negative'. The protein names and interaction-related words were predetermined by human experts and all sentences are manually classified. Consequently, we have got total 1,135 sentences of 'positive' and 569 sentences of 'negative'. Figure 2 shows the examples from positive and negative sentences.

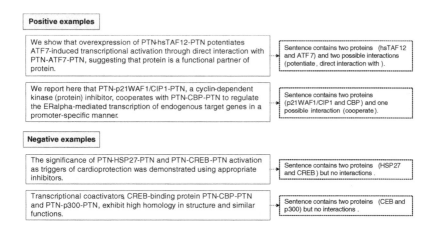

Fig. 2. The examples of 'positive' and 'negative' sentences

4.2   Evaluation Measure

Table 1 presents the labels given as a result of the relationship between a system's output and an answer. Based on the table, the system performance measured as follows:

$$accuracy = \frac{TP + TN}{TP + FP + FN + TN} \cdot 100\%$$

$$precision = \frac{TP}{TP + FP} \cdot 100\%$$

$$recall = \frac{TP}{TP + FN} \cdot 100\%$$

$$F1 - score = \frac{2 \cdot precision \cdot recall}{precision + recall}.$$

Table 1. The labels given as a result of the relationship between a system's output and an answer

		Answer	
		Positive	*Negative*
Test	*Positive*	*TP*	*FP*
Results	*Negative*	*FN*	*TN*

4.3   Protein Interaction Extraction

For experiments, we have used Brill tagger [15] and Collins parser [16] to construct parsing trees. 10-fold cross-validation is performed to evaluate the system performance because the data set is not large enough for a comparative study. We also have generated two different data sets from the original examples. One set contains original sentences with unchanged tags, but the other set is additionally tagged by using new keyword 'PTN' and '-I', which is explained in Section 3.3. The 'PTN' indicates 'protein name' and the '-I' indicates 'interaction-related word'.

We first performed the protein-protein interaction extraction using all 1,704 sentences, which unbalances positive and negative examples. Figure 3 depicts the performance results using tree kernel methods. When $\lambda \leq 0.5$, the tree kernel approach gives high performance in accuracy and F1-score for both data sets. Note that λ in tree kernels has been introduced to scale the relative importance

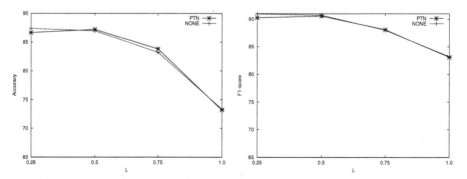

Fig. 3. The performance comparison of the tree kernel methods using all examples

Table 2. The performance comparison of the proposed approach and other methods

Method	Tree Kernel	BOW Kernel	naïve Bayes
Accuracy	87.21	83.96	81.77
F1-score	90.58	88.61	86.71

of tree fragments with their size. Using λ, we can adjust the degree of down-weight according to tree fragments' size. Therefore we can conclude that it is more important to look at the overall structure rather than the detail of the structure, especially for long and complex sentences. However, both data sets do not provide any difference for the tree kernel method. We infer that it occurs from the unbalanced data. The SVM classifier is learned more focusing on positive examples because positive examples are twice more than negative ones, and it causes relatively high recall and blurs other performance factors.

Table 2 presents the performance comparison of our approach and other methods in accuracy and F1-score. It compares with the BOW kernel and the naïve Bayes classifier. The tree kernel performance is the results obtained from 'PTN' and '-I' tag transformation when $\lambda = 0.5$. Our approach shows 87.21% of accuracy and 90.58% of F1-score, while the BOW kernel method shows 83.96% of accuracy and 88.61% of F1-score, and the naïve Bayes classifier shows 81.77% of accuracy and 86.71% of F1-score. Here, we find that the tree kernel methods can provide better performance than typical approaches.

Because of the unbalance issue between the number of positive and negative examples, we have measured the extraction performance using balanced data. Each 569 sentences were randomly chosen from positive and negative examples. Figure 4 presents the performance comparison of our methods using the balanced data. It shows the data set tagged by 'PTN' and '-I' provides better performance than original data set over all λ. It means that the extraction system can improve its performance by using extra tags if protein names and interaction-related words are properly detected and tagged.

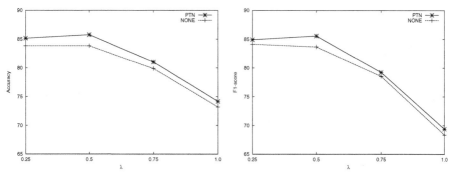

Fig. 4. The performance comparison of the tree kernel methods using randomly selected data

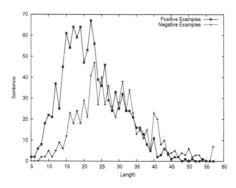

Fig. 5. Number of examples for the sentence length

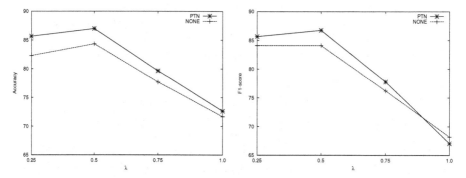

Fig. 6. The performance comparison of the tree kernel methods using randomly selected data, which have similar length

Further, we analyze the number of examples for the sentence length, which
shown in Figure 5. It describes positive examples are relatively short compared
than negative examples. Under same condition of protein and interaction-related
word counts, negative examples have high possibility to be long sentences because
the protein-protein interaction is not involved in the examples. Thus we equally
selected about 440 sentences with similar length from positive and negative examples. Figure 6 presents the performance results using similar length examples.
Like previous results, the best performance is achieved when $\lambda = 0.5$. We can
also think that normalization of word length can be useful to identify protein-
protein interaction although the tree kernel already considers the sentence length
by the parameter λ. It is well known that document length incorporates into the
system performance in IR (Information Retrieval) task.

5   Conclusion

In this paper, we proposed a tree kernel-based method to mine protein-protein
interactions. Our approach transforms each sentence to a tree structure by using

grammatical information, and a support vector machine based on the tree kernel is used to extract the protein-protein interactions. The SVM is learned from the given predefined interaction corpus and interaction patterns. Then it extracts the protein-protein interactions from new sentences.

For experiments, we performed 10-fold cross-validation for 1,135 positive examples and 569 negative examples obtained from PubMed. The experimental results show our approach provides better performance than other methods in accuracy and F1-score. Also, the data set using 'PTN' and '-I' tag transformation supports more accurate extraction, which means that the detection of 'protein names' or 'interaction-related words' is important to improve the performance. It is interesting that the accuracy and the F1-score achieve the highest score when $\lambda \leq 0.5$. It suggests the overall form of tree structure is one of the key points for the extraction performance rather than the detail of structure. However, the tree kernel can be modified to consider sentence length or protein-protein word distance to capture informative factors, which remains as future works.

Acknowledgements

This research was supported in part by the National Research Laboratory Program of the Korea Ministry of Science and Technology and by the Korean Ministry of Education under the BK21-IT Program. The ICT at Seoul National University provided research facilities for this study.

References

[1] Deng, M., Mehta, S., Sun, F., and Chen, T.: Inferring domain-domain interactions from protein-protein interactions. *Genome Research* **12** (2002) 1540–1548

[2] Huang, M., Zhu, X., Hao, Y., Payan, D.G., Qu, K., and Li, M.: Discovering patterns to extract protein-protein interactions from full texts. *Bioinformatics* **20(18)** (2004) 3604–3612

[3] Yakushiji, A., Tateisi, Y., and Miyao, Y.: Event extraction from biomedical parsers using a full parser. In *Proceedings of the 6th Pacific Symposium on Biocomputing* (2001) 408–419

[4] Park, J.C., Kim, H.S., and Kim, J.J.: Bidirectional incremental parsing for automatic pathway identification with combinatory categorical grammar. In *Proceedings of the 6th Pacific Symposium on Biocomputing* (2001) 396–407

[5] Temkin, J.M. and Gilder, M.R.: Extraction of protein interaction information from unstructured text using a content-free grammar. *Bioinformatics* **19(16)** (2003) 2046–2053

[6] Leroy, G. and Chen, H.: Filling preposition-based templates to capture information from medical abstracts. In *Proceedings of the 7th Pacific Symposium on Biocomputing* (2002) 350–361

[7] Pustejovsky, J., Castano, J., Zhang, J., Kotecki, M., and Cochran, B.: Robust relational parsing over biomedical literature: extracting inhibit relations. In *Proceedings of the 7th Pacific Symposium on Biocomputing* (2002) 362–373

[8] Zelenko, D., Aone, C., and Richardella, A.: Kernel methods for relation extraction. *Journal of Machine Learning Research* **3** (2003) 1083–1106

 [9] Lodhi, H., Shawe-Taylor, J., Cristianini, N., and Watkins, C.: Text classification using string kernels. *Journal of Machine Learning Research* **2** (2002) 419–444
[10] Vapnik, V.: *The Nature of Statistical Learning Theory*, Springer, 1995
[11] Cancedda, N., Gaussier, E., Goutte, C., and Renders, J.M.: Word-sequence kernels. *Journal of Machine Learnign Research* **3(6)** (2003) 1059–1082
[12] Collins, M.: New ranking algorithms for parsing and tagging: Kernels over discrete structures, and the voted perceptron. In *Proceedings of 40th Conference of the Associations for Computational Linguistics* (2002) 625–632
[13] Collins, M. and Duffy, N.: Convolution kernels for natural languages. In *Proceedings of the 15th Annual Conference on Neural Information Processing Systems* **14** (2001) 625–632
[14] Hao, Y., Huang, M., and Li, M.: Discovering patterns to extract protein-protein interactions from full texts - part II. *Bioinformatics* **21(15)** (2005) 3294–3300
[15] Brill, E.: Transformation-based error-driven learning and natural language processing: a case study in part-of-speech tagging. *Computational Linguistics* **21(4)** (1995) 543–565
[16] Collins, M.: Head-driven statistical models for natural language parsing. *Doctoral Dissertation*, Dept. of Computer and Information Science, University of Pennsylbania, Philadelphia (1999)

Recognizing Biomedical Named Entities Using SVMs: Improving Recognition Performance with a Minimal Set of Features

Nazife Dimililer and Ekrem Varoğlu

Computer Engineering Department,
Eastern Mediterranean University,
Gazimağusa, Mersin-10, Turkey
{nazife.dimililer, ekrem.varoglu}@emu.edu.tr

Abstract. In this paper, Support Vector Machines (SVMs) are applied to the identification and automatic annotation of biomedical named entities in the domain of molecular biology, as an extension of the traditional named entity recognition task to special domains. The effect of the use of well-known features such as word formation patterns, lexical, morphological, and surface words on recognition performance is investigated. Experiments have been conducted using the train and test data made public at the Bio-Entity Recognition Task at JNLPBA 2004. An F-score of 69.87% was obtained by using a carefully selected combination of a minimal set of features, which can be easily computed from training data without any use of post-processing or external resources.

1 Introduction

There has been tremendous growth in the number of articles in molecular biology and biomedicine lately. This growth has brought up the need for effective and efficient text mining and knowledge discovery in these fields in order to help biologists gather and make use of the knowledge buried in textual documents. Many of these text-mining applications depend on the most crucial first step known as named entity recognition. Bio-entity recognition involves the process of identifying and classifying technical terms in the biomedical domain such as the names of genes, proteins, gene products, cells and organisms' names as well as drugs, chemical compounds, etc. Each term corresponds to a particular concept represented in the text, as a result, the goal of term identification is to recognize the term and capture its underlying meaning.

Even though the progress in Named Entity Recognition (NER) in the newswire domain in the recent years has been satisfactory, automatic identification of named entities in the biomedical domain remains a significantly challenging task. Some of the factors that complicate this task are; use of descriptive naming conventions, use of conjunctions and disjunctions in biomedical entity names, non-standardized naming conventions, use of synonyms, the extensive use of abbreviations, and the fact that some biomedical entity names may be cascaded. Furthermore, new names are constantly being introduced in the domain vocabulary and yet some of these are only used for

E.G. Bremer et al. (Eds.): KDLL 2006, LNBI 3886, pp. 53–67, 2006.
© Springer-Verlag Berlin Heidelberg 2006

relatively short time periods. In addition, there exists ambiguity in the tokenization of biomedical text.

There are three main challenges faced in NER in the biomedical domain that are commonly encountered in many classification problems; forming a more advantageous ensemble of features from existing features, finding new features to aid identification tasks and choosing the most appropriate features for each classification method. The wide variety of features used include, word formation patterns, morphological patterns, part-of-speech (POS), semantic triggers, name alias features, gene sequences, and external resources such as gazetteers. Some of the popular machine learning based classification models used for named entity recognition task in the recent past includes Support Vector Machines (SVMs), Hidden Markov Models (HMMs), Maximum Entropy Markov Models (MEMMs), and Conditional Random Fields (CRFs) [1].

In this paper, we have used a general-purpose chunker named YamCha [2] based on SVMs for automated recognition. SVMs have lately been proven superior to many other machine-learning methods mentioned earlier in the classification of biomedical named entities [3]. The type of features we have used includes, the predicate and the preceding classes as well as lexical features such as, POS, base phrase classes, base NP chunks, morphological patterns, word formation patterns, and surface words constructed from training data. We have considered recall, precision and overall F-scores [4] of systems trained with different types of features and used an ensemble of features based on observations of scores from systems using single features with the aim of maximizing the overall F-score with a minimal set of features. To test the effectiveness of our recognition system, we have used training and test data provided in the Bio-Entity Recognition Task at JNLPBA 2004[1].

In the remainder of this paper, we describe the data set used in our experiments, the specific features investigated, and the SVM-based system used. We present the results obtained and discuss some trends we have observed from our results. Finally, we suggest an ensemble set of features for the NER task, which improves recognition performance.

2   Training and Test Data Used

We trained and tested our systems using the test and training sets provided in the Bio-Entity Recognition Task at the JNLPBA 2004. The training data came from the GENIA corpus v.3.02 [5] and was formed by reducing the number of classes in the corpus from 36 to 5, namely: Protein, DNA, RNA, Cell Line, and Cell Type. The training set is composed of 2000 MEDLINE abstracts collected using the search terms "human", "blood cell", "transcription factor" forming a total number of 472,006 tokens. The test data used was formed specifically for the JNLPBA shared task and it contained 404 abstracts with a total token count of 96,780. The test data was formed by searching a super domain to encourage the generalization properties of the systems in the shared task. Table 1 summarizes the basic statistics of the training data.

---

[1] http://research.nii.ac.jp/~collier/workshops/JNLPBA04st.htm

Table 1. Basic statistics of the training data

		Protein	DNA	RNA	Cell Type	Cell Line	All Entities
Training Data	# of Entities	30269	9533	951	6718	3830	51301
	# of Tokens	55117	25307	2481	15466	11217	109588
Test Data	# of Entities	5067	1056	118	1921	500	8662
	# of Tokens	9841	2845	305	4912	1489	19392

Both training and test data sets used IOB2 representation for chunking where every word is tagged with a class label extended with 'I', representing that the token is inside a named entity chunk, 'O' representing that the token is outside a named entity chunk and 'B', representing that the token is at the beginning of a named entity chunk.

3 Evaluation Methodology

Results are given as F-scores, which is a very common measure based on precision and recall. Precision is defined as a measure of the proportion of the selected items that the system found correctly and recall is defined as the proportion of target items that the system has selected. Precision and recall may be formulated as:

$$\text{Precision} = \frac{TP}{TP + FP} \, , \tag{1}$$

$$\text{Recall} = \frac{TP}{TP + FN} \, , \tag{2}$$

where TP stands for True Positives representing the number of correctly selected entities, FP stands for False Positives representing the number of wrongly selected entities and FN stands for False Negatives representing the number of false rejections. F-score is a value that combines the precision and recall as

$$F - \text{score} = \frac{2 \text{ x Precision x Recall}}{\text{Precision + Recall}} \, . \tag{3}$$

4 Features Used

The features we have used in our study in order to cope with intricacies in the Bio-Entity recognition problem are described below:

- **Predicate:** These are the actual tokens in the training data.
- **Previously Predicted Tags:** These are the predicted tags of the preceding predicates.
- **Morphological features:** Morphological information is considered as an important clue for entity identification in different domains and has been extensively used.

We used different n-grams of the token as features. An n-gram of a token is simply formed by using the last or first n characters of the token.

- **Lexical Features:** These features are grammatical functions of the tokens such as part-of-speech (POS) and phrase position tags. We used three types of lexical features in our experiments.
  - POS Tag: The effect of POS features in NER in the biomedical domains has been tested previously by various researchers and differing views on its effect have been reported [6], [7]. As a result, we decided to test the effect of this feature on the recognition performance of our system. Since the training and test data did not include POS tags, we tagged both data sets using the Geniatagger, which is a POS tagger, trained on both the newswire and biomedical domains.[2]
  - Phrase Tag: We trained an SVM system as a phrase tagger using the newswire domain data. All Noun, Verb, Prepositional, SBAR, Adverb, Adjective phrases etc. were tagged using the IOB2 representation. Then we tagged the train and test data sets using the trained system.
  - Base Noun Phrase Tag: We tagged the train and test data sets with Base Noun Phrases (NP) in IO format by using fnTBLBaseNP[3], which is a BaseNP tagger trained on the newswire data.
- **Word Formation Patterns / orthographic:** These features give information about the capitalization, use of uppercase letters, digits and other word formation information. A close study of the training data revealed that some of the constituents of entities contain special word formation patterns, such as use of a hyphen, words containing uppercase letters (one or many), presence of a Greek letters that may give a clue about its identification. Although many researchers have used orthographic features extensively, to the best of our knowledge, information regarding the contribution of specific orthographic features has not been reported. We have adopted a systematic way of utilizing these patterns based on the representation score of each orthographic feature. We developed an initial list of orthographic features based on previous research as well as our own observation from the training data. For each orthographic feature in the list, we calculated the representation score defined as:

$$\text{Representation Score} = \frac{\text{Number of tokens with the given orthographic feature}}{\text{Total number of all tokens constituting an entity}} \quad (4)$$

This score was calculated for all named entities in the training data as well as the set of tokens that are tagged as OUTSIDE class. We eliminated those orthographic features, which had a representation score higher than 10% in the list of OUTSIDE tokens from the initial list. In this way, we formed a reduced list of orthographic features that possesses more clues for the identification of the entities. The reduced list is used in two different ways:

---

[2] http://www-tsujii.is.s.u-tokyo.ac.jp/GENIA/tagger
[3] http://nlp.cs.jhu.edu/~rflorian/fntbl

- We formed a binary string containing one bit to represent each orthographic feature in the list. The presence of an orthographic feature in a predicate is denoted by a '1' whereas its absence is denoted by a '0'.
- We formed a prioritized list of orthographic features and tagged each token using the first feature in the list that matches it. The prioritized list was formed by ordering the orthographic features in the initial list in decreasing order of their representation score and then modifying the order slightly using some intuition so that the more specific orthographic features precede the general ones. For example a more general property such as "contains upper" would prevent the more specific properties such as "Initial letter capitalized" from ever being used.

Table 2 contains some example orthographic features used in our experiments in decreasing order of representation score among all entity-tagged tokens in the training data.

Table 2. Orthographic Features in Decreasing Order of Representation Score from Top to Down, Left to Right

Orthographic property	Example	Orthographic property	Example
UpperCase	IL-2	UpperOther	2-M
InitCap	D3	LowerUpper	25-Dihydroxyvitamin
TwoUpper	FasL	UpperDigits	AP-1
AlphaOther	AML1/ETO	LowerOther	dehydratase/dimerization
Hyphen	product-albumin	Allupper	DNA, GR, T
Upper_or_Digit	3II	Greek	NF-Kappa, beta
Digits	40	lowerDigits	gp39
AlphaDigit	IL-1beta	startHyphen	-mediated

- **Surface Words:** A pseudo-dictionary was formed for each entity by using the entity tagged tokens (tagged as B or I) in the training data. For each entity, all tokens with the given entity tag were ordered in decreasing order according to the number of its occurrence. To form a pseudo-dictionary for each entity, the top n tokens in each list were chosen, such that the total number of occurrences of these n tokens exceeded a certain percentage of the total number of all tokens of that entity. Four sets of pseudo-dictionaries constituting 50, 60, 70, and 80% of all entity tagged tokens were formed. The 90% case was ignored since this number is very close to almost all the entity tagged tokens in the training data set. The number of distinct tokens and the total number of all tokens in each pseudo-dictionary are given in Table 3. Each token in the training and test set was tagged with a 5-bit binary string where each bit represents a different entity. The presence of a token in a pseudo-dictionary of an entity is marked with a '1' and its absence is marked with a '0'. For example the token 'cell' appears in the pseudo-dictionary of protein, cell type and cell line entity, therefore it is tagged with the string '11010'.

Table 3. Number of Tokens in each Pseudo-dictionary

Percentage	Entity	Number of unique entries in dictionary	Total number of tokens
50%	Protein	103	27550
	Cell Line	14	5533
	DNA	61	12616
	Cell Type	8	7571
	RNA	13	1215
60%	Protein	198	32954
	Cell Line	36	6721
	DNA	116	15120
	Cell Type	19	9229
	RNA	27	1459
70%	Protein	387	38534
	Cell Line	109	7885
	DNA	219	17499
	Cell Type	41	10815
	RNA	62	1735
80%	Protein	774	43862
	Cell Line	270	8976
	DNA	475	20079
	Cell Type	99	12450
	RNA	135	1999

5   System Description

The system we used throughout this study is a general-purpose text chunker named Yet Another Multipurpose Chunk Annotator- YamCha[4] that uses TinySVM[5]. SVM is a powerful machine learning method that has been used successfully in Named Entity Recognition tasks in biomedical as well as newswire domains [3], [8].   SVM classifiers find the optimal hyper-plane that separates the positive and negative data samples with the maximum margin and uses this hyper-plane to classify the data as positive or negative. YamCha takes in the training and test data and transforms them into feature vectors, which can be used by the SVM.

An example input to YamCha is shown in Fig. 1. The file contains one token on each line. There may be a number of features separated by white space next to each token. The last column on a line is the correct tag of the token. In the example shown here, the token to be classified is shown at position 0. The correct tag of the token is shaded. YamCha uses a context window, which contains both static and dynamic components.   The static content of the context window includes preceding and following tokens and the respective features to be used for classification. The dynamic component of the context window may only include the estimated tags of the preceding tokens.

---

[4] http://chasen.org/~taku/software/yamcha
[5] http://chasen.org/~taku/software/TinySVM

	Token	Feature (POS)	Feature (Suffix)	Feature (Prefix)	Tag
Position:-4	total	JJ	al	tot	O
Position:-3	content	NN	nt	con	O
Position:-2	of	IN	of	of	O
Position :-1	T	NN	T	T	B-cell_type
Position: 0	lymphocytes	NNS	es	lym	I-cell_type
Position: +1	was	VBD	as	was	O
Position:+2	decreased	VBN	ed	dec	O
Position:+3	1.5-fold	RB	ld	1.5	O
Position:+4	in	IN	in	in	O

Fig. 1. Context Window

There are several parameters of YamCha, which affect the number of support vectors. These parameters are the dimensionality of the polynomial kernel, range of the context window, direction of parsing, and the method for solving a multi-class problem.

6   Discussion and Results

We used the evaluation script provided with the training and test data sets at the JNLPBA shared task to compute the recall, precision and F-scores for the identification of entities. The script computes three sets of precision, recall and the F-score values. For each named entity, these scores are calculated for the entities correctly identified at the left boundary, entities correctly identified at right boundary and entities correctly identified at both boundaries. The same set of scores is also computed for the overall, or object, identification performance.

Table 4. Object Identification Scores of the Baseline System

Full			Left			Right		
Recall	Precision	F-Score	Recall	Precision	F-Score	Recall	Precision	F-Score
0.6275	0.6574	0.6421	0.6669	0.6987	0.6825	0.7087	0.7425	0.7252

6.1   Base Line System

In order to analyze the effect of different features and parameters on the recognition performance we have set up a base line system. For this purpose, we trained our system using only the tokens in the training data and predicted entity tags. The baseline system was trained in forward parse direction using second degree polynomial kernel with one-vs.-all method. The context window size is -2 to 2. The performance of the baseline system is shown in Table 4.

In the remainder of this study, all experiments were trained using the one-vs.-all approach. We studied the effect of different features and parse direction on the object identification performance. To show the general behavior of the trained systems, we computed the average scores of all experiments with similar characteristics. Our results are presented in the following sections.

6.2 Effect of Parse Direction

To study the effect of the parsing direction on performance, we performed similar experiments using both forward (from left to right) and backward (from right to left) directions with different features and their various combinations as well as different window sizes. Table 5 shows the average scores of these experiments for object identification.

Table 5. Effect of Parse Direction on Object Identification

Parse Direction	Full			Left			Right		
	Recall	Precision	F-Score	Recall	Precision	F-Score	Recall	Precision	F-Score
Forward	0.6521	0.6530	0.6523	0.6918	0.6928	0.6920	0.7292	0.7302	0.7294
Backward	0.6685	0.6813	0.6745	0.7051	0.7187	0.7115	0.7493	0.7638	0.7561

It can be seen that backward parsing causes a significant increase in the precision and recall values of both left and right object boundaries, resulting in an increase of 2.22% in the object full F-score. When backward parsing is used, the left boundary F-score is improved by 1.95% whereas right boundary F-score is improved by 2.67%. The precision values are increased by 2.58% on the left boundary and by 3.36% on the right boundary. On the other hand, the improvement in the recall values turned out to be lower both for the left and right boundaries, 1.32% and 2.02% respectively. It can be deduced from these results that backward parsing improves precision scores more than recall scores and furthermore the improvement in the overall identification performance is mainly due to a performance increase on the right boundary which can easily be explained by the right to left parsing direction.

6.3 Effect of Morphological Features

We have used different n-grams as morphological features in our experiments. Both suffixes and prefixes up to n=4 were formed for use as features in our system. We wanted to check the effect of each feature type individually and as a result, we performed tests using single features. Table 6 shows the effect of using prefixes only, suffixes only and feature combinations of suffix and prefixes as features on object identification performance. The results given are average values from tests in both parsing directions. Results clearly indicate an improvement in F-score from the use of morphological features. It is interesting to note that the use of suffixes results in higher recall values compared to precision values where as the reverse is true when prefixes are used. This observation suggests that the combination of both features should improve the overall of F-score for object identification.

Table 6. Effect of Morphological Features on Object Identification

Morph. Features Used	Full			Left			Right		
	Recall	Precision	F-Score	Recall	Precision	F-Score	Recall	Precision	F-Score
Prefix	0.6448	0.6513	0.6479	0.6843	0.6912	0.6876	0.7251	0.7323	0.7286
Suffix	0.6547	0.6484	0.6514	0.6936	0.6868	0.6901	0.7363	0.7293	0.7327
Combined	0.6575	0.6504	0.6539	0.6968	0.6893	0.6930	0.7389	0.7310	0.7348

6.4 Effect of Lexical Features

We trained systems with single lexical features as well as different combinations containing lexical features. The lexical features we used were POS tag, Base Noun Phrase tags in IO format, and Phrase Type tag in IOB2 format. The study involving the single lexical features was repeated with different context window sizes since it is expected that the neighboring tokens and tags will be very useful in classification of the current token for this feature. We also tested the effect of combining two lexical features together. These experiments involve using POS feature either with the Base Noun Phrase feature or with the Phrase Type feature. The average results of experiments in both parsing directions are shown in Table 7.

Table 7. Effect of Lexical Features on Object Identification

Lexical Features Used	Full			Left			Right		
	Recall	Precision	F-Score	Recall	Precision	F-Score	Recall	Precision	F-Score
Single	0.6346	0.6751	0.6541	0.6724	0.7154	0.6931	0.7100	0.7553	0.7318
Combined	0.6553	0.6663	0.6607	0.6946	0.7062	0.7003	0.7308	0.7430	0.7368

The first row shows the effect of using only one lexical feature, and the second row shows the effect of using combinations of lexical features only. Even though the BaseNP and Phrase Type tagging depends on the POS tag, the combination of these features slightly improves performance. More specifically, it is observed that combining lexical features results in an increase in recall values and a less significant drop in precision values. Consequently, combination slightly improves performance of both the left boundary and the right boundary F-scores resulting in a minor improvement of 0.66% in the full F-score.

6.5 Effect of Word Formation Patterns

A careful examination of the training data reveals that the constituents of the entities have some special orthographic patterns such as containing a hyphen or a mixture of upper case letters and numbers or Greek letters. We designed experiments with single orthographic features based on this intuition. The main difficulty in using these features is in choosing which feature to use since the list of features reported in literature can be quite long and furthermore their performance can differ significantly. For example, some of the experiments using features such as "contains upper case letters" gave satisfactory results (object full F-score 0.6546) but some others such as "contains Greek letter" (object full F-score 0.6438) had less improvement.   One approach would be to use as many features as possible, but this would increase the number of features significantly. Furthermore, our studies revealed that not all orthographic features mix well. As discussed earlier our approach is to use two types of more sophisticated orthographic features as a single feature.   In the first method, we used a binary string where each bit represents the presence or absence of a specific orthographic feature.   The second sophisticated single orthographic feature we used was based on a prioritized list of word formation patterns.   The average values from experiments using all three methods in both parse directions are shown in Table 8.

Table 8. Effect of orthographic features on object identification performance

Orthographic Features Used	Full			Left			Right		
	Recall	Precision	F-Score	Recall	Precision	F-Score	Recall	Precision	F-Score
Simple	0.6569	0.6593	0.6579	0.6953	0.6979	0.6964	0.7397	0.7425	0.7409
Priority Based	0.6802	0.6562	0.6680	0.7191	0.6936	0.7061	0.7606	0.7337	0.7468
Binary String	0.6848	0.6546	0.6694	0.7226	0.6907	0.7063	0.7658	0.7320	0.7485

It can be seen that the sophisticated orthographic feature based on the use of a binary string improves the performance slightly better than the sophisticated orthographic feature based on a prioritized list. It is interesting to note that when simple orthographic features are used precision scores turn out to be slightly higher than recall scores. However when sophisticated orthographic features are used the full object recall scores turns out to be higher than precision scores up to almost 3%. When the performance of the simple and sophisticated orthographic features are compared, a decrement of less than 0.47% in the precision scores of sophisticated orthographic features is observed; nevertheless, this drop is compensated by a much significant improvement of 2.79% in the recall scores. This results in an overall improvement of 1.15% in the full object F-score when the sophisticated orthographic feature based on the binary string is used in comparison to the simple orthographic feature.

6.6   Effect of Surface Word Features

We formed experiments using the surface word feature in order to test the effect of using surface words.   In order to check the effect of the size of the pseudo-dictionary on identification performance we formed four sets of pseudo-dictionaries.   For each entity tag, we used a certain percentage of all tokens tagged as that entity (marked as B or I) to form a pseudo-dictionary. These pseudo-dictionaries were then used to form the surface word feature, which is a single feature in the form of a binary string where each bit represents an entity class. A bit representing the entity class is set to '1' if the token is in the pseudo-dictionary, which belongs to that entity class.

Table 9 shows the recall, precision and F-score values of all systems trained using a single surface word feature. The results presented are the average of systems using backward and forward parsing. It is observed that the use of surface words with any pseudo-dictionary size improves both recall and precision scores compared to the baseline system and that the improvement on precision is more pronounced. It is also seen that the average F-scores using different dictionary sizes remain within 0.73%, suggesting that dictionary size is not very significant. Nevertheless, the improvement on F-scores suggests that using a dictionary-based approach is worth considering.

Table 9. Effect of Surface Word Feature on Object Identification Scores

Pseudo-dictionary size	Full			Left			Right		
	Recall	Precision	F-Score	Recall	Precision	F-Score	Recall	Precision	F-Score
50%	0.6324	0.6699	0.6506	0.6702	0.7098	0.6894	0.7153	0.7577	0.7358
60%	0.6339	0.6736	0.6531	0.6714	0.7134	0.6918	0.7168	0.7616	0.7385
70%	0.6348	0.6765	0.6550	0.6723	0.7164	0.6936	0.7174	0.7645	0.7402
80%	0.6271	0.6698	0.6477	0.6650	0.7102	0.6868	0.7090	0.7572	0.7323

We also examined the effect of excluding stop words from the surface word feature. The stop word list used in our experiments is from Rijbergen [9]. Two main approaches were used for this purpose: The first approach was to eliminate the stop words from the list of available tokens of each entity and then perform the calculations on dictionary coverage using the new list. Results of this experiment are shown in Table 10 as SW exp1. The second approach was to add a new bit to represent whether or not the token is in the stop word list without modifying the original pseudo-dictionaries. The presence of a '1' denotes that the word is in the stop word list and the presence of a '0' denotes that it is not. This new bit was added in two different ways. In the first method, the new bit was added as the least significant bit of the binary string to form a single 6-bit pseudo-dictionary. The result of this experiment is shown as SW exp2a in Table 10. Finally, we designed experiment SW exp2b where the bit representing the presence of a stop word is added as an additional feature after the 5-bit pseudo-dictionary feature. We performed these experiments using a pseudo-dictionary of 60% since the size of the dictionary proved to be of less importance. The parse direction was backward. Unfortunately, excluding the stop words had a negative effect on the performance of the system. This may be due to the fact that, there are many named entities in the training data that contain stop words in their name.

Table 10. Effect of Excluding Stop Words on Object Performance

Features Used	Full			Left			Right		
	Recall	Precision	F-Score	Recall	Precision	F-Score	Recall	Precision	F-Score
Pseudo-Dic. 60%	0.6411	0.6829	0.6613	0.6799	0.7243	0.7014	0.7241	0.7714	0.7470
SW exp1	0.6403	0.6795	0.6593	0.6799	0.7215	0.7001	0.7263	0.7708	0.7479
SW exp 2a	0.6405	0.6833	0.6612	0.6762	0.7213	0.6980	0.7219	0.7701	0.7452
SW exp 2b	0.6400	0.6782	0.6586	0.6771	0.7175	0.6967	0.7224	0.7655	0.7433

6.7 Combination of Features

We combined the features discussed in the previous sections based on our observations of their performance when used as single features. The strategy adopted was to combine the features in such a way that they complement each other's strengths and weaknesses in precision and recall values. Since backward parsing improved F-scores significantly, we trained all systems using a combination of features with backward parsing. Furthermore the context window size was kept fixed identical to the baseline system for a fair comparison. It was observed that some specific combinations of feature types do not have a significant improvement in performance. However, our results suggest that careful combination of features proves to be useful. The average full object identification results of experiments where feature combinations significantly improved performance are given in Table 11. Here, the first row shows the performance of the baseline system.

Table 11. Average Full Object Identification Scores using Combination of Features: All Systems

Lexical	Morpho-logical	Surface words	Word Formation Pattern	Full Object Identification		
				Recall	Precision	F-Score
				0.6275	0.6574	0.6421
x				0.6399	0.6729	0.6558
x	x			0.6744	0.6682	0.6712
x	x	x		0.6844	0.6669	0.6755
x	x	x	x	0.7006	0.6791	0.6897

Although a clear indication of improvement in recall, precision, and F-scores can be easily deduced from he average scores presented, the success of our system can be more clearly seen when we compare the performance of best systems for each set of combinations. Table 12 shows these results.

Table 12. Full Object Identification Scores using Combination of Features: Best Systems

Lexical	Morpho-logical	Surface words	Word Formation Pattern	Full Object Identification		
				Recall	Precision	F-Score
				0.6275	0.6574	0.6421
x				0.6649	0.6769	0.6708
x	x			0.6946	0.6844	0.6895
x	x	x		0.6974	0.6893	0.6933
x	x	x	x	0.7058	0.6918	0.6987

Moreover, we have found that a combination involving all feature types discussed previously has a significant improvement in F-scores. It can be seen that, using this combination of features, recall, precision and F-scores increase by 7.83%, 3.44%, and

5.66% respectively compared to the baseline system. The significance of this particular combination is that it uses only 5 features, a single feature from each feature type (2 for morphological) as discussed before.

Finally, we discuss the identification performance of our best system on different entity tags compared to the baseline system. Table 13, shows the full object identification scores for each entity tag.

Table 13. Full Identification Scores: Baseline System vs. Best System

Entity	Recall		Precision		F-score	
	Baseline	Best	Baseline	Best	Baseline	Best
Protein	0.6623	0.7578	0.6555	0.6860	0.6589	0.7201
Cell Line	0.5020	0.5620	0.5389	0.5009	0.5202	0.5297
DNA	0.5833	0.6638	0.6318	0.7131	0.6066	0.6876
Cell Type	0.5945	0.6304	0.7164	0.7694	0.6498	0.6930
RNA	0.5932	0.6864	0.6140	0.6639	0.6034	0.6750

It can be deduced from Table 13 that using a combination of features improves the F-score values for all entities. The maximum increase in full identification F-score is obtained for DNA, RNA and protein entities whereas the increase for cell line entity is minimal. The F-score values of the best system for DNA, RNA and protein has improved by 7.16%, 8.1% and 6.12% respectively. The behavior of the best system considering recall and precision values varies amongst entities. The highest improvements in full recall values have been for the protein entity by 9.55%, and RNA entity by 9.32%. Our best system improves the recall scores of protein, cell line, and RNA entities significantly more than their precision scores. However, the cell type entity behaves differently; there is a more significant improvement of 5.3% in precision as opposed to recall of 3.59%. Furthermore, it is interesting to note that although there is a considerable improvement in the recall value of the cell line entity; its precision is worsened compared to the baseline line system. Another interesting observation is that the improvement on recall and precision values of the DNA entity are very balanced, 8.05% and 8.13% respectively.

A similar pattern of scores can be seen in both the left and right boundary identification as expected. The results are shown in the Tables 14 and 15 for left and right boundaries respectively.

Table 14. Left Boundary Identification Scores: Baseline System vs. Best System

Entity	Recall		Precision		F-score	
	Baseline	Best	Baseline	Best	Baseline	Best
Protein	0.7186	0.8078	0.7111	0.7312	0.7148	0.7676
Cell Line	0.5300	0.596	0.5699	0.5312	0.5492	0.5617
DNA	0.6061	0.6638	0.6564	0.7131	0.6302	0.6876
Cell Type	0.6039	0.6398	0.7277	0.7808	0.6600	0.7033
RNA	0.6017	0.7034	0.6228	0.6803	0.6121	0.6917

Table 15. Right Boundary Identification Scores: Baseline System vs. Best System

Entity	Recall		Precision		F-score	
	Baseline	Best	Baseline	Best	Baseline	Best
Protein	0.7312	0.8307	0.7236	0.7519	0.7274	0.7893
Cell Line	0.5900	0.6760	0.6344	0.6025	0.6111	0.6371
DNA	0.6610	0.7292	0.7159	0.7833	0.6873	0.7553
Cell Type	0.7069	0.7184	0.8519	0.8767	0.7227	0.7897
RNA	0.7034	0.7797	0.7281	0.7541	0.7155	0.7667

The best system shows the highest improvements on DNA, RNA and protein entities at the boundaries. The improvements of F-scores on the left boundary for these entities are 7.5%, 7.96%, and 5.28% respectively. The improvements of F-scores on the right boundary for the same entities are 6.8%, 5.12% and 6.19% respectively. Even though the F-score of the RNA entity is improved slightly more than the F-score of the DNA entity on the left boundary, DNA has a more significant improvement on the right boundary and thus it has a higher full object F-score increase. The smallest amount of improvement in full object identification F-score is seen for cell line entity where the precision score of our best system is lower than the precision score of the baseline system. Despite this weakness, the best system improves the recall values of the cell line entity to give a noticeable improvement in F-scores of 1.25 % on the left boundary and 2.57% on the right boundary.

7 Conclusion

In this paper, we presented an SVM based system for the named entity recognition task in the biomedical domain. We discussed the effect of different features on performance. We have aimed to achieve a high performance through a careful combination of a minimal set of features by performing experiments with single features and combining systems in such a way that they compensate each other's weaknesses. Our best system achieves a full object F-score of 69.87%. This performance is lower than the performance of the two best performing systems [3], [10] at the JNLPBA 2004 Named Entity Recognition Task. However, the two systems, which outperform our best system, use more features and rely on post-processing and/or the use of external resources. The system presented here, uses no external sources and no post-processing methods. The features used in all of our experiments are easily computed from the training data, which minimizes the time required to prepare the data for training. We argue that a careful selection of the features used for training will reduce the size of the optimal feature vector resulting in a reduction in processing time; a very important phenomenon for SVM based classifiers.

Our work will concentrate on designing an ensemble classifier system for the named entity recognition task based on an automatic intelligent selection of the systems discussed in this paper.

Acknowledgements

This work is supported by the Ministry of Education and Culture of TRNC.

References

1. Duda R. O., Hart P. E., Stork D. G.: Pattern Classification. John-Wiley and Sons (2001)
2. Kudo T, Matsumoto Y.: Chunking with Support Vector Machines. Proceedings of Second Meeting of North American Chapter of the Association for Computational Linguistics (NAACL) (2001) 192-199
3. Zhou G., Su J.: Exploring Deep Knowledge Resources in Biomedical Name Recognition. Proceedings of the International Joint Workshop on Natural Language Processing in Biomedicine and its Applications (JNLPBA-2004). Geneva, Switzerland (2004) 96-99
4. Manning C.D., Schutze H.: Foundations of Statistical Language Processing. MIT Press, Cambridge, Massachusetts (1999)
5. Ohta T., Tatishi Y., Mima H., Tsujii J.: The GENIA corpus: an annotated research abstract corpus in the molecular biology domain. Human Language Technologies Conference (HLT-2002). San Diego (2002) 489-493
6. Collier N., Takeuchi K.: Comparison of Character-level and part of speech features for name recognition in biomedical texts. Journal of Biomedical Informatics 37 (2004) 423-435
7. Zhou G., Zhang J., Su J., Shen D., Tan C.: Recognizing Names in biomedical texts: a machine learning approach. Bioinformatics (2003) 1178-1190
8. Mayfield J., McNamee P., Piatko C.: Named Entity Recognition using Hundreds of Thousands of Features. Proceedings of CoNLL-2003. Edmonton, Canada (2003) 184-187
9. van Rijsbergen C.J.: Information retrieval. 2nd edn. Butterworths, London (1979)
10. Finkel J., Dingare S., Nguyen H., Nissim M., Sinclair G., Manning C.: Exploiting Text for Biomedical Entity Recognition: From Syntax to the Web. Proceedings of the International Joint Workshop on Natural Language Processing in Biomedicine and its Applications (JNLPBA-2004). Geneva, Switzerland (2004) 88-91

Investigation of the Changes of Temporal Topic Profiles in Biomedical Literature

Wei Huang[1,2], Shouyang Wang[2], Lean Yu[2], and Hongtao Ren[3]

[1] School of Management, Huazhong University of Science and Technology,
WuHan, 430074, China
[2] Institute of Systems Science, Academy of Mathematics and Systems Sciences,
Chinese Academy of Sciences, Beijing, 100080, China
{whuang, sywang, yulean}@amss.ac.cn
[3] School of Knowledge Science, Japan Advanced Institute of Science and Technology,
Asahidai 1-1, Tatsunokuchi, Ishikawa, 923-1292, Japan
hongtao@jaist.ac.jp

Abstract. We represent research themes by the temporal topic profiles based on MeSH terms from MEDLINE citations. By comparing the differences of the temporal profiles for the same topic at the two different periods, we find that the temporal profiles for a topic at the new period may result from three kinds of concepts replacements of the temporal profiles at the old period, namely broad replacement, parallel replacement and narrow replacement. Such findings provide new ways to generate potential relationships from the current biomedical literature.

1 Introduction

The idea of discovering new relationships from a bibliographic database was first introduced by Swanson [1]. Swanson describes an approach that discovers relationships between concepts that are logically related but not bibliographically related, i.e., do not co-occur in any document. The general idea is that two entities A and C might be related if A co-occurs in some document with intermediate entity B, and B co-occurs in some document with C [2, 3]. While Stephens et al., also used co-occurrence data to postulate gene interactions, they went beyond simple frequency based counts and also considered how frequently the gene term (or its synonyms) occurs in the documents [4]. Weeber et al. replicated Swanson and Smalheiser's experiments on Raynaud's disease and fish oils by limiting the interesting phrases extracted to MeSH terms [5, 6]. Jenssen et al analyzed the titles and abstracts of MEDLINE records to look for co-occurrence of gene symbols [7]. The main advantage of this method in comparison with the kernel document method is that it avoids the difficulty of selecting an appropriate kernel document. However, this method cannot identify genes that are functionally related, but are not mentioned together in any MEDLINE abstract. Such implicit relationships between genes are inherently more interesting in the context of mechanism/pathway discovery by computation. Srinivasan and Rindflesch presented a text mining application that

E.G. Bremer et al. (Eds.): KDLL 2006, LNBI 3886, pp. 68–77, 2006.

exploits the MeSH subheadings combinations in the MEDLINE citations [8]. The process begins with a user specified pair of subheadings. Co-occurring concepts qualified by the subheadings are regarded as being conceptually related and thus extracted. A parallel process using SemRep, a linguistic tool, also extracts conceptually related concepts pairs from the title of MEDLINE citations. The pairs extracted via MeSH and the pairs extracted via SemRep are compared to yield a high confidence subset. These pairs are then combined to project a summary associated with the selected subheading pairs. The limitation in their work is that they need to refine the output of the summarization step since the UMLS tends to be incomplete. In addition, entries that are at different levels of generality confound the output. Zhu et al. presented the feasibility of using co-occurrence of MeSH terms to find some useful relationships in Medical literature using association rules mining [9]. Narayanasamy et al developed a system called "Trans-Miner" to find associations among biological objects such as genes, proteins, and drugs by mining the MEDLINE database of the scientific literature [10]. Wren et al. first constructed a network of tentative relationships between "objects" of biomedical research interest (e.g. genes, diseases, phenotypes, chemicals) by identifying their co-occurrences within all electronically available MEDLINE citations. Relationships shared by two unrelated objects were then ranked against a random network model to estimate the statistical significance of any given grouping [11, 12]. They demonstrated that an analysis of shared relationships scored against a random network model has the potential to elucidate novel and interesting relationships not documented within MEDLINE, but rather based upon information contained therein. However, there are shortcomings in the use of this method: First, there is the problem of "uninteresting" relationships. To some extent, this will be user-dependant. Objects that share many relationships may indeed have a relationship themselves, but the nature of their relationship may be such that it would not be considered interesting or worth investigating. Second, ascertaining the nature of the implied relationship by examining the shared relationships is time-consuming according to their experiments. Finally, work still needs to be done on better establishing relationships, beyond what they have done in scoring the probability that a co-occurrence was meaningful. For example, the method asserts that a relationship is known when two objects have been mentioned together within the same abstract, and unknown if they have not. While this may be a good generalization, two objects may have been co-mentioned several times and yet the overall nature of their relationship, or certain aspects thereof, remains unknown.

In the previous work, the researchers have not considered to measure the relationships of objects by other ways. The implicit relationships are inferred by just combining the co-occurrences of objects. Is there any new ways to generate potential relationships from the current biomedical literature? In order to answer the question, we need to find the connections of the research themes during the different periods. Our contribution is to represent research theme in a structured form called temporal topic profile, and compare the profiles of the same topic at two different periods. The remainder of this paper is organized as follows. Section 2 describes the methods to judge the relationships of the two MeSH terms. Section 3 builds temporal topic profiles. In Section 4, we conduct the experiments to compare the profiles of the six topics at the two periods. Finally, conclusions are given in Section 5.

2 Judge the Relationships of the Two MeSH Terms

Since the late 1800s, the U.S. National Library of Medicine (NLM) has used its own list of terms for medicine. This vocabulary is used by the NLM to catalogue books, other library materials, and to index articles for inclusion in health related databases including MEDLINE. This preferred list of terms is known as Medical Subject Headings(MeSH). The goal of MeSH is to provide a reproducible partition of concepts relevant to biomedicine for purposes of organization of medical knowledge and information. MeSH vocabulary is utilized to retrieve information about a medical topic. For example, in MEDLINE, MeSH terms are used to conduct specific subject searches. MeSH terminology provides a controlled or consistent way of retrieving information that may use different terminology for the same concept.

In addition to its alphabetical listing, MeSH terminology is organized hierarchically. This hierarchical listing is referred to as tree structures. The tree structures provide an effective way to browse broad and narrow MeSH terms in order to find appropriate concepts to search. The tree structures consist of 15 broad subject categories (see Figure 1) category A for anatomic, category B for organisms, C for diseases, D for drugs and chemicals, etc. which are further subdivided into more specific subcategories. Within each subcategory, MeSH terms are arrayed hierarchically from most general to most specific in up to eleven hierarchical levels. When searching MeSH, the term being searched will be displayed within a hierarchy of broader (more general) headings above it, and narrower (more specific) headings below it. MEDLINE citations are indexed with the most specific MeSH terms available. The user may select to search the most appropriate MeSH heading for the topic.

Anatomy [A]
Organisms [B]
Diseases [C]
Chemicals and Drugs [D]
Analytical, Diagnostic and Therapeutic Techniques and Equipment [E]
Psychiatry and Psychology [F]
Biological Sciences [G]
Physical Sciences [H]
Anthropology, Education, Sociology and Social Phenomena [I]
Technology and Food and Beverages [J]
Humanities [K]
Information Science [L]
Persons [M]
Health Care [N]
Geographic Locations [Z]

Fig. 1. Top level of MeSH tree structures

The U.S. National Library of Medicine makes a hierarchical arrangement MeSH terms with their associated tree numbers available in an electronic file. Figure 2 shows sample text from MeSH Trees. Each MeSH term is followed by its tree number, which shows its location in the tree. The tree numbers are the formal computable representation of the hierarchical relationships. Using the tree number associated with each MeSH term, we can judge the relationships of MeSH terms in the hierarchical structure, MeSH tree.

Reptiles;B02.833

    Alligators and Crocodiles;B02.833.100

    Dinosaurs;B02.833.150

    Lizards;B02.833.393

       Iguanas;B02.833.393.500

    Snakes;B02.833.672

       Boidae;B02.833.672.250

       Colubridae;B02.833.672.280

Fig. 2. Sample text from MeSH tree

In order to judge the relationships of the two MeSH terms, we introduce the following three functions:

(1) Function $T(n_i)$ returns the MeSH term corresponding to the tree number n_i. For example, $T(\text{B02.833.100})=$ Alligators and Crocodiles.

(2) Function , $L(n_i)$ returns the length of the tree number n_i .For example, $L(\text{B02.833.100})=11$.

(3) Function $F(n_i, l)$ returns a substring of the tree number n_i from the first character of n_i and the length of the substring is l .

For example, $F(\text{B02.833.100}, 7)=$ B02.833, $F(\text{B02.833.100}, 3)=$ B02.

We can judge the relationships of the two MeSH terms in MeSH tree according to their corresponding tree numbers by using the above tree functions. Let n_i and n_j be two tree numbers; then $T(n_i)$ and $T(n_j)$ are the two corresponding MeSH terms.

2.1 Super-Relationship

If

$$L(n_j) + 4 = L(n_i),\tag{1}$$

$$F(n_i, L(n_i) - 4) = n_j,\tag{2}$$

Then $T(n_j)$ is a super-concept of $T(n_i)$.

For example, "Reptiles" is a super-concept of "Alligators and Crocodiles", because the tree number of "Reptiles" is B02.833 and the tree number of "Alligators and Crocodiles" is B02.833.100, which satisfy

$$L(\text{B02.833}) + 4 = L(\text{B02.833.100})\tag{3}$$

$$F(\text{B02.833.100}, 11\text{-}4) = \text{B02.833}\tag{4}$$

2.2 Sibling Relationship

If

$$L(n_j) = L(n_i) \tag{5}$$

$$F(n_j, L(n_j) - 4) = F(n_i, L(n_i) - 4) \tag{6}$$

Then $T(n_j)$ is a sibling concept of $T(n_i)$.

For example, "Dinosaurs" is a sibling concept of "Alligators and Crocodiles", because the tree number of "Dinosaurs" is B02.833.150 and the tree number of "Alligators and Crocodiles" is B02.833.100, which satisfy

$$L(B02.833.150) = L(B02.833.100) \tag{7}$$

$$F(B02.833.150, 11\text{-}4) = F(B02.833.100, 11\text{-}4) \tag{8}$$

Similarly, "Lizards" and "Snakes" are also sibling concepts of "Alligators and Crocodiles".

2.3 Sub-relationship

If

$$L(n_j) - 4 = L(n_i) \tag{9}$$

$$F(n_j, L(n_j) - 4) = n_i \tag{10}$$

Then $T(n_j)$ is a sub-concept of $T(n_i)$.

For example, "Iguanas" is a sub-concept of "Lizards", because the tree number of "Iguanas" is B02.833.393.500 and the tree number of "Lizards" is B02.833.393, which satisfy

$$L(B02.833.393.500) - 4 = L(B02.833.393) \tag{11}$$

$$F(B02.833.393.500, 11\text{-}4) = B02.833.393 \tag{12}$$

Similarly, "Boidae" and "Colubridae" are two sub-concepts of "Snakes".

3   Building Temporal Topic Profiles

We build temporal topic profiles by identifying a relevant subset of documents for a specific period from MEDLINE using just the MeSH term. The temporal profile for topic T_i at period t are weighted vectors of MeSH term as follows:

$$P(T_i, t, w) = \{w_{i,t,1} m_{i,t,1}, w_{i,t,2} m_{i,t,2}, \ldots, w_{i,t,j} m_{i,t,j}, \ldots\} \tag{13}$$

where w is the set threshold value to filter the MeSH terms whose weight is smaller than w; $m_{i,t,j}$ is the jth MeSH term appearing in the set of MEDLINE citations on topic T_i at period t; $w_{i,t,j}$ is the corresponding weight of $m_{i,t,j}$. Weight $w_{i,t,j}$

represents the relative importance of MeSH term $m_{i,t,j}$ to the topic T_i. Weight $w_{i,t,j}$ may be computed using any appropriate weighting scheme, such as mutual information and log likelihood. Below we use the TF*IDF (term frequency * inverse document frequency) [13] weighting scheme. If w is larger, there are fewer MeSH terms in topic temporal profiles.

Topics profiled may be in free text format, i.e., not limited to the MeSH terms. Topics may be as simple as single word (e.g. Tylenol) or as complex as collection of words specified by users.

We divide MEDLINE citations about a topic T_i into two segments according to the publication dates, and build the corresponding temporal profiles $P(T_i, t_{old}, w)$ and $P(T_i, t_{new}, w)$, respectively. We can get some useful knowledge by comparing the topic temporal profiles $P(T_i, t_{old}, w)$ and $P(T_i, t_{new}, w)$.

In this paper, we just focus on the new appearing MeSH terms in topic profile $P(T_i, t_{new}, w)$. The change of weights for the MeSH terms appearing in both $P(T_i, t_{old}, w)$ and $P(T_i, t_{new}, w)$ will be discussed in the future research. Therefore, let $w = 0$, and the temporal profile for topic T_i at period t can be simply represented with a set of MeSH terms as follows:

$$P(T_i, t) = \{m_{i,t,1}, m_{i,t,2}, \ldots, m_{i,t,j}, \ldots\} \tag{14}$$

For example, the temporal profile for topic "Raynaud's disease" at period $t = 1969 - 1985$ is as follow:

$$P(\text{Raynauds disease}, 1969 - 1985) =$$
$$\{\text{blood platelets, elbow joint, eosinophils, erythrocytes, \ldots}\} \tag{15}$$

Set $P(T_i, t_{new}) - P(T_i, t_{old})$ contains the MeSH terms that are in $P(T_i, t_{new})$ and are not in $P(T_i, t_{old})$. Our goal is to find the relationship of MeSH terms in the sets $P(T_i, t_{new}) - P(T_i, t_{old})$ and $P(T_i, t_{old})$.

4   Experiments Analysis

In order to reduce noise and speed up calculation, we only consider major MeSH terms of each MEDLINE citation. Major MeSH terms associated with each citation serve as important concepts that represent the main topics of each citation. The co-occurrence of two major MeSH terms in a MEDLINE citation implies a specific relationship, while the co-occurrence of two non-major MeSH terms or major MeSH term and non-major MeSH term in a MEDLINE citation might be meaningless or too broad. For example, Gene Expression and Alleles are appearing as the non-major MeSH terms in the MEDLINE citation in Figure 3. However, it is trivial to implicitly connect Gene Expression with Alleles by their co-occurrence, because all genes have alleles, even if it is not explicitly specified.

PMID- 8550811

......

TI - Tumor necrosis factor alpha-308 alleles in multiple sclerosis and optic neuritis.

......

AB - Tumor necrosis factor-alpha (TNF-alpha), a proinflammatory cytokine, is be-
lieved to play an important role in multiple sclerosis (MS) pathogenesis.

......

......

MH - Alleles

MH - Base Sequence

MH - Gene Expression

MH - Genotype

...

MH - Multiple Sclerosis/*genetics/ immunology

MH - Optic Neuritis/*genetics/immunology

MH - Phenotype

MH - Polymerase Chain Reaction

MH - Polymorphism (Genetics)

MH - Promoter Regions (Genetics)/genetics

MH - RNA, Messenger/immunology

MH - Support, Non-U.S. Gov't

MH - Tumor Necrosis Factor/*genetics

......

SO - J Neuroimmunol 1995 Dec 31;63(2):143-7.

Fig. 3. An example of MEDLINE citations

We divide the MEDLINE citations into two segments according to the publication
date, namely old segment (t_{old}: 1990-1995) and new segment (t_{new}: 1996-1999).
The two periods are just chosen for examples without any specific purpose. For topic
T_i, we build two temporal profiles $P(T_i, t_{old})$ and $P(T_i, t_{new})$ from MEDLINE citations on topic T_i in the two segments, respectively. We examine how many the
MeSH terms in the set $P(T_i, t_{new}) - P(T_i, t_{old})$ are super-concepts, sibling concepts,
sub-concepts of MeSH terms in the set $P(T_i, t_{old})$.

Table 1 shows the experiment results of the six topics. Let's take the first topic
temporal arteritis in Table 1 as an example. There are 210 MeSH terms in the set
$P(\text{temporal arteritis}, t_{new}) - P(\text{temporal arteritis}, t_{old})$. Among the 210 MeSH terms,
10% are super-concepts of the MeSH terms in the set $P(\text{temporal arteritis}, t_{old})$; 41% are
sibling concepts of the MeSH terms in $P(\text{temporal arteritis}, t_{old})$; 22% are sub-concepts
of the MeSH terms in the set $P(\text{temporal arteritis}, t_{old})$. For the topic melanoma, there are
975 MeSH terms in the set $P(\text{melanoma}, t_{new}) - P(\text{melanoma}, t_{old})$. Among the 975
MeSH terms, 15% are super-concepts of the MeSH terms in the set $P(\text{melanoma}, t_{old})$;
65% are sibling concepts of the MeSH terms in $P(\text{melanoma}, t_{old})$; 42% are sub-

concepts of the MeSH terms in the set $P(\text{melanoma}, t_{old})$. The sum of 15%, 66% and 42% is larger than 100%, because each MeSH term appears in at least one place in the MeSH tree and may appear in as many additional places as may be logically appropriate, so it may have more than one tree number. A MeSH term can be super-concept, sibling concept and sub-concept of different MeSH terms at the same time. For example, some of the 975 MeSH terms are super-concepts of a MeSH terms and sibling concepts of another MeSH term in the set $P(\text{melanoma}, t_{old})$ at the same time.

Table 1. The changes of temporal profiles for the six topics

topic T_i	$P(T_i, t_{new}) - P(T_i, t_{old})$	super-concept	sibling concept	sub-concept
temporal arteritis	210	10%	41%	22%
melanoma	975	15%	65%	42%
chondrodysplasia punctata	38	18%	42%	29%
charcot-marie-tooth disease	170	11%	45%	15%
noonan syndrome	77	10%	46%	13%
ectodermal dysplasia	198	7%	44%	17%

The experiment results show that sibling concepts accounts for the largest percent, around half of the MeSH terms in the set $P(T_i, t_{new}) - P(T_i, t_{old})$; sub-concepts and super-concepts are in the second and third place in the rank for the percents of the MeSH terms in the set $P(T_i, t_{new}) - P(T_i, t_{old})$. It indicates that a topic temporal profile's changes may result from the three types of concepts replacements, namely broad replacement, parallel replacement and narrow replacement. Broad replacement is to replace a concept with its super-concept. Parallel replacement is to replace a concept with its sibling concept. Narrow replacement is to replace a concept with its sub-concept. In the descending order of percentage of concepts replacement, parallel replacement, narrow replacement and broad replacement are ranked in the first, second and third place, respectively. It is consistent with researchers' normal thinking way when they extend existing research themes. For example, researchers want to discover new treatments for a disease A. By reviewing the literature on disease A, researchers have known some treatments associated with disease A. For example, drug B is related to disease A. Then, the drugs related to B may serve as potentially new treatments for disease A. Siblings of drug B, e.g., drug C, are first considered, because they are similar to drug B. Drug C may have some properties which are the same as drug B. On the other hand, drug C has other different properties, which may have interesting effect on disease A, for example positive or negative. It is also interesting to consider the sub-concepts and super-concepts of drug B.

According to the results, we may design new way to generate potential relationships from the current biomedical literature. We can first represent the current findings in biomedical literature with structured forms, and then change some parts of the structured forms by using the above three concept replacements. It should be noted that such process are implemented by the interaction with the researchers in the bio-medical fields, because their background knowledge and research interests will help focus on the more interesting changes.

5   Conclusions

In this paper, we build MeSH term-based temporal topic profiles from MEDLINE citations and investigate the changes of temporal profiles for a topic at two different periods. We find that the temporal profiles for a topic at new periods may result from three kinds of the three types of concepts replacements, namely broad replacement, parallel replacement and narrow replacement. In the descending order of percentage of concepts replacement, parallel replacement, narrow replacement and broad re-placement are ranked in the first, second and third place, respectively. Such findings actually provide new ways to generate potential relationships from the current bio-medical literature.

Acknowledgements

This work is partially supported by National Natural Science Foundation of China (NSFC No. 70221001) and the Key Research Institute of Humanities and Social Sciences in Hubei Province-Research Center of Modern Information Management.

References

1. Swanson, D. R.: Fish oil, Raynauds Syndrome, and Undiscovered Public Knowledge. Per-spectives in Biology and Medicine, **30** (1986) 7-18
2. Swanson, D. R.: On the Fragmentation of Knowledge, the Connection Explosion, and As-sembling Other People's Ideas. Bulletin of the American Society for Information Science and Technology, **27** (2001) 12-14
3. Swanson, D. R., Smalheiser, N. R. & Bookstein, A.: Information Discovery from Com-plementary Literatures: Categorizing Viruses as Potential Weapons. Journal of the Ameri-can Society for Information Science and Technology, **52** (2001) 797-812
4. Stephens, M., Palakal, M., Mukhopadhaya, S., Raje, R. & Mostafa, J.: Detecting Gene Re-lations from MEDLINE Abstracts. Proceedings of Pacific Symposium on Biocomputing, Hawaii, January 3-7, (2001) 483-496
5. Weeber, M., Vos, R., Klein, H. & de Jong-van den Berg, L. T. W.: Using Concepts in Lit-erature-Based Discovery: Simulating Swanson's Raynaud-fish Oil and Migraine-Magnesium Discoveries. Journal of the American Society for Information Science and Technology, **52** (2001) 548-557
6. Weeber, M., Vos, R., Klein, H., de Jong-van den Berg, L. T. W., Aronson, A. R. & Molema, G. Generating Hypotheses by Discovering Implicit Associations in the Litera-ture: a Case Report of a Search for New Potential Therapeutic Uses for Thalidomide. Journal of the American Medical Informatics Association, **10** (2003) 252-259

7. Jenssen, T. K., Laegreid, A., Komorowski, J. & Hovig, E.: A Literature Network of Human Genes for High-Throughput Analysis of Gene Expression. Nature Genetics, **28** (2001) 21-28
8. Srinivasan, P. & Rindflesch, T.: Exploring Text Mining from MEDLINE. Annual Conference of the American Medical Informatics Association (AMIA 2002), (2002) 722-726
9. Zhu, A. L., Li, J. & Leong, T. Y.: Automated Knowledge Extraction for Decision Model Construction: a Data Mining Approach. Proceedings of the American Medical Informatics Association (AMIA) Annual Fall Symposiu, (2003) 758-762
10. Narayanasamy, V., Mukhopadhyay, S., Palakal, M. & Potter, D. A.: TransMiner: Mining Transitive Associations among Biological Objects from Text. Journal of Biomedical Science, **11** (2004) 864-73
11. Wren, J. D., Bekeredjian, R., Stewart, J. A., Shohet, R. V. & Garner, H. R.: Knowledge Discovery by Automated Identification and Ranking of Implicit Relationships. Bioinformatics, **20** (2004) 389-398
12. Wren, J. D. & Garner, H. R.: Shared Relationship Analysis: Ranking Set Cohesion and Commonalities within a Literature-Derived Relationship Network. Bioinformatics, **20** (2004) 191-198
13. Sparck J. K.: A Statistical Interpretation of Term Specificity and Its Application in Retrieval. Journal of Documentation, **28** (1972) 111–121

Extracting Protein-Protein Interactions in Biomedical Literature Using an Existing Syntactic Parser

Hyunchul Jang[1], Jaesoo Lim[1], Joon-Ho Lim[1], Soo-Jun Park[1],
Seon-Hee Park[1], and Kyu-Chul Lee[2]

[1] Bioinformatics Research Team,
Electronics and Telecommunications Research Institute (ETRI),
Gajeong-Dong, Yuseong-Gu, Daejeon, Republic of Korea 305-350
{janghc, jslim, joonho.lim, psj, shp}@etri.re.kr
[2] Department of Computer Engineering, Chungnam National University,
Gung-Dong, Yuseong-Gu, Daejeon, Republic of Korea 305-764
kclee@cnu.ac.kr

Abstract. We are developing an information extraction system for life science literature. We are currently focusing on PubMed abstracts and trying to extract named entities and their relationships, especially protein names and protein-protein interactions. We are adopting methods including natural language processing, machine learning, and text processing. But we are not developing a new tagging or parsing technique. Developing a new tagger or a new parser specialized in life science literature is a very complex job. And it is not easy to get a good result by tuning an existing parser or by training it without a sufficient corpus. These all are another research topics and we are trying to extract information, not to develop something to help the extracting job or else. In this paper, we introduce our method to use an existing full parser without training or tuning. After tagging sentences and extracting proteins, we make sentences simple by substituting some words like named entities, nouns into one word. Then parsing errors are reduced and parsing precision is increased by this sentence simplification. We parse the simplified sentences syntactically with an existing syntactic parser and extract protein-protein interactions from its results. We show the effects of sentence simplification and syntactic parsing.

1 Introduction

Many of the previous researchers have extracted information in biomedical text by matching the sentences with predefined patterns or rules [1,2,3,4,5,6]. These approaches can be effective on limited types of events in a limited domain. The workload of preparing patterns for extraction would be expensive if we expand our attentions to texts of other domains or to a wider scope of event [7].

Huang *et al.* proposed a method for automatically generating patterns and extracting protein interactions [8,9]. Bunescu *et al.* showed that various rule induction methods are able to identify protein interactions with higher precision than manually-developed rules [10]. Ramani *et al.* used a set of 230 Medline abstracts manually tagged for both proteins and interactions to train an interaction extractor [11]. But,

E.G. Bremer et al. (Eds.): KDLL 2006, LNBI 3886, pp. 78–90, 2006.
© Springer-Verlag Berlin Heidelberg 2006

machine learning techniques are also limited by the quality and extent of the training sets used to train the algorithms.

Natural language processing techniques have been widely applied for information extraction in the biomedical domain. Many researchers have used shallow or partial parsing methods, like POS tagging or chunking, because of the difficulty of full parsing [12].

Park *et al.* proposed a full parsing method, using bidirectional incremental parsing with combinatory categorical grammar (CCG) [13]. This method first localizes the target verbs and then scans the left and right neighborhood of the verb. The recall and precision rates of the system were reported to be 48% and 80%, respectively. Temkin *et al.* introduced a method for extracting protein, gene and small molecule interactions from unstructured text [10]. By utilizing a lexical analyzer and context free grammar (CFG), they demonstrate that efficient parsers can be constructed for extracting these relationships with a recall rate of 63.9% and a precision rate of 70.2%. These methods are inherently complicated and domain sensitive, requiring many resources.

Yakushiji *et al.* introduced an information extraction system using a full parser that analyzes the whole structure of sentences [14]. They partially solved the problems of full parsing of inefficiency, ambiguity, and low coverage by introducing the preprocessors, and proposed the use of modules that handles partial results of parsing for further improvement. They converted the surface form of sentences to an intermediate canonical form using a general-purpose, domain independent parser and grammar. Then event information is extracted by domain-specific mapping rules.

Daraselia *et al.* presented an information extraction system based on a full-sentence parsing approach [15]. Their system contains three modules, preprocessor aimed to identify and tag various biomedical domain-specific concepts, NLP engine constructing the set of alternative semantic sentence structures and information extraction module acting as a domain-specific filter for these structures.

Rinaldi *et al.* proposed a method for discovery of interactions between genes and proteins from the scientific literature, based on a complete syntactic analysis of the GENIA corpus [16,17]. They extracted relations from domain corpora based on a full parsing of the documents and on a set of rules that map syntactic structures into the relevant relations.

2   Methods

Parsing a sentence is analyzing the sentence and determining its structure. Morphological knowledge concerns how words are constructed from more basic meaning units called morphemes, where a morpheme is the primitive unit of meaning in a language. Syntactic knowledge concerns how words can be put together to form correct sentences and determines what structural role each word plays in the sentence [12,18].

Although it is not simple to parse biomedical sentences syntactically with a parser not tuned in biomedical domain or it is hard to develop a new parser for biomedical domain, we aim to parse sentences syntactically to extract protein-protein interactions because syntactic relations can be recognized simply.

We agree that a modular architecture that separates NLP and information extraction into different modules is efficient [15]. The NLP module deals with the domain-independent sentence structure decomposition, while the information extraction module can be reconfigured towards different tasks [7].

We apply the result of a parser in forms of the Penn Treebank syntactic tags [19]. Fig. 1 (a) is an example sentence and (b) shows the parsing result for it. Fig. 2 shows the syntactic tag tree structure and how we extract an interaction between two proteins by traversing the tree. It is similar to find a path between two leaf nodes.

(a)

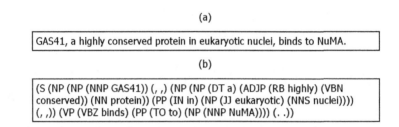

(b)

Fig. 1. (a) An original sentence (b) Parsing result

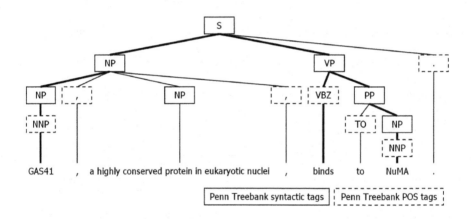

Fig. 2. A Penn Treebank tag tree of a sentence

In Fig. 2, the sentence presents in the form of NP+VP. 'GAS41' represents the NP phrase, 'binds' and 'NuMA' represent the VBZ and PP phrase in VP phrase. This is not a passive form and there is no negative expression. So, 'GAS41' is the subject of the 'binds' event and 'NuMA' is the object.

To achieve the above, we must parse given target sentences to syntactic tag tree like Fig. 2. Many existing full parsers, not tuned to biomedical domain, frequently fail to parse, or their parsed results are often incorrect. These are caused by that most sentences in biomedical literature are syntactically complex or words in sentences are tagged incorrectly. The sentence of Fig. 3 is an example. This sentence has 43 tokens when the parentheses are tokenized and the minus symbols are not tokenized.

To define the mechanism underlying signal transducer and activator of transcription (STAT) protein recruitment to the interleukin 10 (IL-10) receptor the STAT proteins activated by IL-10 in different cell populations were first defined using electrophoretic mobility shift assays.

Fig. 3. An original sentence

For this reason we need a well-tuned parser in biomedical literature but we don't have it. We could find good trainable full parsers but there is no available syntactically tagged corpus in biomedical domain for learning. Building a corpus of proper size is not a simple job at all. The accomplishment of a corpus is closely related to the parser's performance. Full parsing in one domain is another good research topic. So we are focusing on well-use of an existing syntactic parser.

We introduce our method to parse sentences syntactically and to extract interaction information from them. Fig. 4 shows the flowchart.

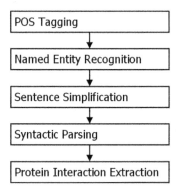

Fig. 4. Flowchart

2.1 Tagging Sentences

The first step to syntactic parsing and extracting protein-protein interactions is tagging sentences morphologically. There are two major reasons. One reason is that tagging results of a tagger are better than a full parser because a tagger can be trained with a morphologically tagged corpus but there is no proper corpus for a full parser in biomedical domain. So if the parser can receive the POS-tagging results, it can produce better parsing results. The other reason is that morphological tags are good features for named entity recognition.

The sentence of Fig. 3 is tagged like Fig. 5.

2.2 Making Sentences Simple

Biomedical sentences are generally complex. One reason is that named entities in biomedical texts are usually not simple and consist of many words those have various morphological tags. It makes difficult to parse biomedical texts. One named entity can be divided into different phrases and it makes the structure collapse. So we make them simpler.

To/TO define/VB the/DT mechanism/NN underlying/VBG signal/NN
transducer/NN and/CC activator/NN of/IN transcription/NN (/(STAT/NN)/)
protein/NN recruitment/NN to/TO the/DT interleukin/NN 10/CD (/(IL-
10/NN)/) receptor/NN ,/, the/DT STAT/NN proteins/NNS activated/VBN
by/IN IL-10/NN in/IN different/JJ cell/NN populations/NNS were/VBD first/RB
defined/VBN using/VBG electrophoretic/JJ mobility/NN shift/NN assays/NNS ./.

Fig. 5. A POS-tagged sentence

Yakushiji *et al.* introduced two preprocessors that resolve the local ambiguities in sentences to improve the efficiency [7]. One is a term recognizer that glues the words in a noun phrase into one chunk so that the parser can handle them as if it is one word. The other is a shallow parser that reduces the lexical ambiguity.

We use our named entity recognizer to solve this problem. First, we substitute recognized named entities with one word like Table 1. We made our named entity recognizer to extract all proteins tagged in the Yapex corpus. Second, we substitute noun phrases, actually nouns with one word like Table 1 instead of gluing the words in a noun phrase into one chunk. Third, we remove parenthesis phrases (PPR) those are not a part of a named entity.

Table 1. Substitution list

	Original Words (Proteins)	Substituted Words
Named Entity Substitution	signal transducer and activator of transcription	NEA
	STAT	NEB(removed)
	interleukin 10 (IL-10) receptor	NEC
	STAT	NED
	IL-10	NEE
Noun Phrase Substitution	protein recruitment	NPA
	cell populations	NPB
	mobility shift assays	NPC

To/TO define/VB the/DT mechanism/NN underlying/VBG NEA/NNP NPA/NN
to/TO the/DT NEC/NNP ,/, the/DT NED/NNP proteins/NNS activated/VBN
by/IN NEE/NNP in/IN different/JJ NPB/NN were/VBD first/RB defined/VBN
using/VBG electrophoretic/JJ NPC/NN ./.

Fig. 6. A simplified sentence

Then we can have a more simplified sentence. The sentence above is changed like Fig. 6. This sentence now has 27 tokens. Then the parser can process this sentence correctly.

Additionally, in case of 'protein/protein interaction', this phrase must be a noun phrase. But this phrase is tokenized to 'protein / protein interaction' and can be divided into two NP or other phrases. To prevent this problem, we substitute 'and' for '/', '-', '+', and '*'.

2.3 Full Parsing Sentences

The parser returns syntactically tagged sentences as shown in Fig. 7 and their tree structure as shown in Fig. 8.

(S (S (VP (TO To) (VP (VB define) (NP (DT the) (NN mechanism)) (NP (NP (VBG underlying) (NNP NEA) (NN NPA)) (PP (TO to) (NP (DT the) (NNP NEC)))))))) (, ,) (NP (NP (DT the) (NNP NED) (NNS proteins)) (VP (VBN activated) (PP (IN by) (NP (NP (NNP NEE)) (PP (IN in) (NP (JJ different) (NN NPB))))))) (VP (VBD were) (ADVP (RB first)) (VP (VBN defined) (S (VP (VBG using) (NP (JJ electrophoretic) (NN NPC)))))) (. .))

Fig. 7. Results of the parser: Penn Treebank syntactic tags of a sentence

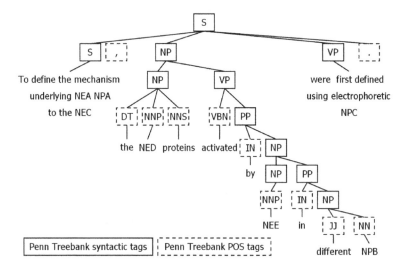

Fig. 8. A Penn Treebank syntactic tag tree of a sentence

Then, our extractor can analyze the whole syntactic structure of sentences. Instead of converting to some templates or structures, we use syntactic tags and trees of sentences. Our rules can be simple and small because the syntactic tag set have less number of tags than the POS tag set. The structural complexities of sentences are simplified into the tree hierarchy.

2.4 Extracting Protein-Protein Interactions

It is not simple to decide whether extracted paths between leaf nodes of a syntactic tree structure are meaningful relations. But if two leaf nodes are proteins, it is easier to decide whether there is a relation or not.

First, the extractor finds NP tags and then checks whether NP is a part of the following 3 cases: NP+VP, NP+PP and NP+CC+NP. 95.4% of 215 interactions are one of the 3 cases. The other sentences belongs the following two cases. One is like 'is-a' semantically, for an example, 'JAB has recently been identified as a regulator of JAK2 phosphorylation and activity by binding phosphorylated JAK2 and inducing its degradation.' This sentence involves 'JAB phosphorylates JAK2' information. And another one is: JJ+NNP, for an example, 'CD38-associated Lck'.

Table 2. Syntactic structures of protein-protein interactions

NP+VP	NP+PP	NP+CC+NP	Others	Total
89	87	29	10	215
41.4%	40.5%	13.5%	4.6%	100%

2.4.1 NP+VP

In Fig. 2, the sentence has NP and VP. 'GAS41' is the first noun of the first NP in the top NP. The extractor looks the first NP in the top NP and finds the first noun, NNP in it. It finds the verb, VBZ in the VP and 'binds' is extracted. Finally, it looks PP after VBZ and finds NP. 'NuMA' is extracted from NP. In the same manner, 'MDM2', 'inhibits' and 'p53' are extracted from the example in Fig. 9.

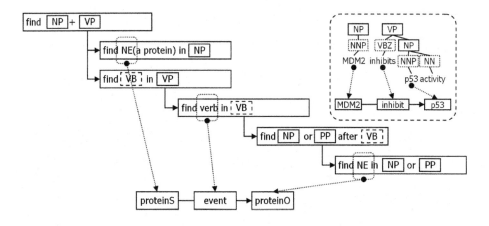

Fig. 9. Flowchart of extraction from NP+VP

2.4.2 NP+PP

We manually defined each type of required PP phrases. So the extractor keeps searching one more PP phrase after extracting 'activation' and 'ERK2'.

2.4.3 NP+CC+NP

In all cases, a NNP-tagged protein is extracted as a subject or an object only when it is the first noun in NP and this NP is the first NP in its parent NP or PP. If a protein or a NP follows CC, they and their parent are available as a subject or an object. Negative expressions can be extracted from RB or DT tags in any phrase.

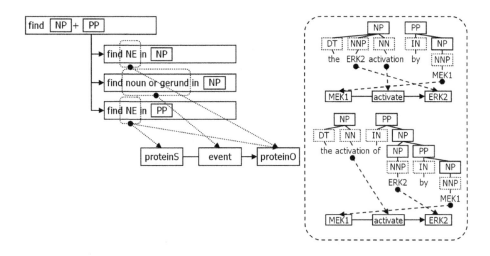

Fig. 10. Flowchart of extraction from NP+PP

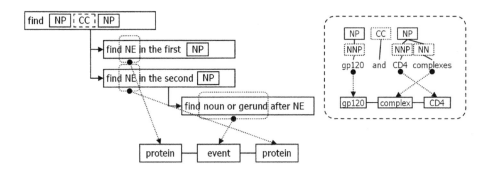

Fig. 11. Flowchart of extraction from NP+CC+NP

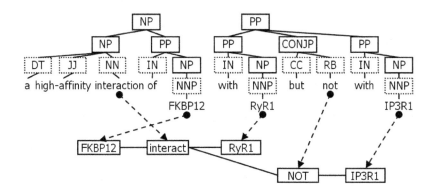

Fig. 12. Extraction of complex and negative information

3 Implementation

We used the Brill's transformation based part-of-speech tagger[1] [20], trained with the GENIA corpus[2] [16].Its precision is 98.35% after training with GENIA corpus and 83.73% with WSJ corpus.

Our named entity recognizer extracts 39 types of named entities including protein, DNA, RNA. But we set it to extract proteins only and enhanced its rules to recognize all proteins in the Yapex testing corpus. When it extracts other types of named entities, the parser can get a change to parse more number and more precisely. Oppositely, when it can't recognize some proteins in real world, the parser may fail more. An important thing is that one missed protein can cause to lose one interaction.

We actually use 'NAMEDENTITYA' and 'NOUNPHRASEA' as the substituted strings instead of 'NEA' and 'NPA' and we modified lexicons to tag substituted named entity words as a NNP and to tag substituted noun phrase words as a NN.

We used the Stanford Parser[3] version 1.4 with probabilistic context free grammar (PCFG).

A small number of biologists marked interactions among the proteins that already tagged in the Yapex testing corpus. We used it as the answer set and the number of the tagged interactions is 215.

4 Experimental Results

We selected Yapex corpus to evaluate our method. The Yapex corpus has been used for the purpose of evaluating named entity recognition methods. But it is neither complex nor difficult to decide the answer set of protein-protein interactions because proteins are already tagged. Yapex corpus consists of 99 abstracts for training and 101 abstracts for testing. We evaluated with the 101 testing abstracts.

4.1 Full Parsing Sentences

Yapex testing corpus has 962 sentences including abstract titles. The number of sentences that have more than two protein names is 532. The parser processed 439 sentences and could not handle 93 sentences. The percentage of parsed sentences is 82.5% and the average number of tokens per a sentence is 24.97. The percentage of failed sentences is 17.5% and the average number of tokens per a sentence is 49.07.

After sentence simplification, the parser can parse 62 sentences more and 31 of 93 sentences are left to fail. The average number of tokens is 26.15 in 501 sentences and 53.38 words in 31 sentences.

We did not evaluate the precision of parsed results but 62 sentences (11.7%) could be parsed after simplification. It means that sentences can be parsed more correctly.

---

[1] Eric Brill's Home Page: http://www.cs.jhu.edu/~brill/RBT1_14.tar.Z
[2] GENIA corpus: http://www-tsujii.is.s.u-tokyo.ac.jp/~genia/topics/Corpus/
[3] The Stanford Natural Language Processing Group: http://www-nlp.stanford.edu/software/lex-parser.shtml

Table 3. Parsing before and after sentence simplification

Sentence Simplification	Full Parsing	
	Success	Fail
Before	439(82.51%)	93(17.48%)
After NES	455(85.52%)	77(14.47%)
After NES+NPS	474(89.09%)	58(10.90%)
After NES+NPS+PPR	501(94.17%)	31(05.82%)

4.2 Extracting Protein-Protein Interactions

We extracted protein-protein interactions from the selected 532 sentences. If a sentence include more than one interaction, all interactions were counted as answers and our system tried to extract all.

We did not evaluate our method without the sentence simplification. Extracted protein names can be scattered over the syntactic tree and our interaction extraction method do not handle this problem.

Table 4. Recall and precision: (a) for 4 events: interact, associate, bind and complex. (b) for all events. We'll talk about the precision value (100.0%) in 5. Discussion.

Type	TP+FN	TP	FP	Recall (%)	Precision (%)
		(a)			
Interact	56	49	2	87.5	96.1
Associate	12	8	0	66.7	100.0
Bind	53	42	1	79.2	97.7
Complex	24	23	0	95.8	100.0
Total for 4	145	122	3	84.1	97.6
		(b)			
Phosphorylate	12	2	0	16.7	100.0
Activate	19	17	0	89.5	100.0
Other	39	28	1	71.8	96.6
Total	215	169	4	78.6	97.7

Table 5. Missed interactions

Type	Missed	(%)
Parsing Fail	3	6.5
Parsing Error	9	19.6
Anaphora	3	6.5
Semantic	31	67.4

Table 4 shows the recall and precision of extraction with the sentence simplification. We calculated that the value of recall is TP/(TP+FN)*100 and the value of precision is FP/(TP+FP)*100. TP indicates the number of interactions extracted correctly by our method, TP indicates the total number of interactions correctly extracted and tagged in the corpus, FN indicates the total number of interactions not extracted but tagged in the corpus and TP+FP indicates the total number of interactions extracted correctly or wrongly by our method.

The recall and precision for the 4 events (Interact, Associate, Bind, Complex) are 84.1% and 97.6%. We extracted more event types additionally: phosphorylate, activate, inhibit, induce, encode, regulate, mediate, stimulate, etc. The total recall and precision are 78.6% and 97.7%. Both negative and passive expressions are included in the answer conditions.

The event 'phosphorylate' returns a lower recall, because sentences containing phosphorylating information are more complicated than others in the Yapex testing corpus. Those sentences need to be handled semantically. For examples, our system didn't understand that 'leads to phosphorylation of' means 'phosphorylate' in this sentence 'Receptor activation by the haematopoietic growth factor proteins interleukin 5 (IL-5) and granulocyte-macrophage colony-stimulating factor (GM-CSF) leads to phosphorylation of JAK2 as a key trigger of signal transduction.' and 'the ability of c-Abl' means 'c-Abl does' in this sentence 'We find that p73 is a substrate of the c-Abl kinase and that the ability of c-Abl to phosphorylate p73 is markedly increased by gamma-irradiation.'

Among the missed 46 interactions, 12 interactions are caused by parsing fail or error. Parsing fail means that the parser can't and parsing error means that it does not correctly. Only 3 interactions tagged in Yapex testing corpus include anaphora terms and we didn't analyze them yet.

Most missed interactions are caused by semantic problems. Our extractor cannot understand semantic relations and syntactic tags don't indicate them. The following sentences are the examples: 'Interaction cloning and characterization of RoBPI, a novel protein binding to human Ro ribonucleoproteins.', 'We analyzed the abilities of fibrillins and LTBPs to bind latent TGF-beta by their 8-Cys repeats.', and 'In vitro GAS41 bound to the C-terminal part of the rod region of NuMA.'

The false positively extracted interactions are caused by parsing error like: 'We conclude that the two NF-IL6 sites mediate induction of IL-1 beta in response to the stimuli LAN, LPS, and TNF-alpha.' The parser thought that 'the two NF-IL6 sites mediate TNF-alpha'.

5   Discussion

We evaluated our method from Yapex testing corpus. There are only 215 interactions and so the recall and precision value may be not accurate so much. We will evaluate using another way such as Ono *et al*'s approach.

Another factor of results is that we have supposed that all proteins are known and recognized. If we miss some of them, we may lose some relations. And we have used a syntactic full parser and our results are greatly influenced by its performance.

Our extraction method has some errors except parsing problems. One is from anaphoric terms. The following sentence is an example: 'Deletion of the binding site from MEK1 reduced its phosphorylation by ERK2, but had no effect on its phosphorylation by p21-activated protein kinase-1 (PAK1).'

Another is from semantic terms. 'We analyzed the abilities of fibrillins and LTBPs to bind latent TGF-beta by their 8-Cys repeats.' Syntactic parsers cannot analyze that 'abilities' are 'binding TGF-beta'. 'The N-terminal end of nebulin interacts with tropomodulin at the pointed ends of the thin filaments.' 'N-terminal end' is a part of a protein. 67.4% of missed events are caused by this reason and percentage of events need semantic processing is 14.5%.

6 Conclusion

We have introduced a method to extract protein-protein interactions from biomedical literature automatically. The basic idea of our approach is that sentences in biomedical literature will be simplified after phrase substitution and a normal full parser can parse these simplified sentences even though the parser is not tuned to biomedical sentences. Then, our system reads the result of the parser and extracts the interactions.

We extracted various types of protein-protein interactions using an existing syntactic parser and got 78.6% recall and 97.7 precision. It is difficult to compare with different techniques by a lack of a standard common corpus for reporting recall and precision [21]. But we concluded that the syntactic parsing is effective.

References

1. Ono, T., Takagi, T.: Automated Extraction of Information on Protein-Protein Interactions from the Biological Literature. Bioinformatics Vol. 17 no. 2 (2001) 155-161
2. Sekimizu, T., Park, H. S., Tsujii, J.: Identifying the Interaction between Genes and Gene Products Based on Frequently Seen Verbs in Medline Abstracts. Genome Informatics Workshop (1998) 62-71
3. Friedman, C., Kra, P., Yu, H., Krauthammer, M. and Rzhetsky, A.: GENIES: a natural-language processing system for the extraction of molecular pathways from journal articles. Bioinformatics Vol. 17 Suppl. 1 (2001) S74-S82
4. Ng, S., Wong, M.: Toward Routine Automatic Pathway Discovery from On-line Scientific Text Abstracts. Genome Informatics Workshop (1999) 104-112
5. Thomas, J., Milward, D., Ouzounis, C., Pulman, S. and Carroll, M.: Automatic Extraction of Protein Interactions from Scientific Abstracts. Proceedings of the 5th Pacific Symposium on Biocomputing (2000) 541-552
6. Wong, L.: PIES, a Protein Interaction Extraction System. Proceedings of the 6th Pacific Symposium on Biocomputing (2001) 520-531
7. Yakushiji, A., Tateisi, Y., Miyao, Y., Tsujii, J.: Event extraction from biomedical papers using a full parser. Proceedings of the 6th Pacific Symposium on Biocomputing (PSB 2001) 408-419
8. Huang, M., Zhu, X., Hao, Y., Payan, D. G., Qu, K., Li, M.: Discovering Patterns to Extract Protein-Protein Interactions from Full Texts. Bioinformatics Vol.20 no. 18 (2004) 3604-3612

9. Hao, Y., Zhu, X., Huang, M., Li, M.: Discovering Patterns to Extract Protein-Protein Interactions from the Literature: Part II. Bioinformatics Vol.21 no. 15 (2005) 3294-3300

10. Bunescu, R., Ge, R., Kate, R. J., Marcotte, E. M., Mooney, R. J., Ramani, A. K., Wong, Y. W.: Comparative Experiments on Learning Information Extractors for Proteins and the Interactions. Journal of Artificial Intelligence in Medicine 33 (2004) 139-155

11. Ramani, A. K., Bunescu, R. C., Mooney, R. J. and Marcotte, E. M.: Consolidating the set of known human protein-protein interactions in preparation for large-scale mapping of the human interactome. Genome Biology Vol. 6, Issue 5 (2005) R40.1-11

12. Sekimizu, T., Park, H.S., Tsujii, J.: Identifying the Interaction between Genes and Gene Products based on Frequently Seen Verbs in Medline Abstracts. Genome Informatics Workshop (1998) 62-71

13. Park, J. C.: Using Combinatory Categorial Grammar to Extract Biomedical Information. IEEE Intelligent Systems, Special Issue on Intelligent Systems in Biology (2001) 62-67

14. Temkin, J.M., Gilder, M.R.: Extraction of Protein Interaction Information from Unstructured Text Using a Context-Free Grammar. Bioinformatics 19 (2003) 2046-2053

15. Daraselia, N., Yuryev, A., Egorov, S., Novichkova, S., Nikitin, A. and Mazo, I.: Extracting human protein interactions from MEDLINE using a full-sentence parser. Bioinformatics Vol. 20 no.5 (2004) 604-611

16. Kim, Jin-Dong, Ohta, T., Tateisi, Y. and Tsujii, J.: GENIA corpus - a semantically annotated corpus for bio-textmining. Bioinformatics Vol. 19(suppl. 1) (2003) i180-i182

17. Rinaldi, F., Schneider, G, Kaljurand, K., Dowdall, J, Andronis, C., Persidis, A., Konstanti, O.: Mining relations in the GENIA corpus. Proceedings of the Second European Workshop on Data Mining and Text Mining for Bioinformatics (2004) 61-68

18. Allen, J.: Natural Language Understanding 2nd Edition, The Benjamin/Cummings Publishing Company, Inc. (1995)

19. Marcus, M. P., Santorini, B., Marcinkiewicz, M. A.: Building a large annotated corpus of English: the Penn Treebank. Computational Linguistics Vol. 19 (1994) 313-330

20. Brill, E.: Transformation-Based Error-Driven Learning and Natural Language Processing: A Case Study in Part-of-Speech Tagging. Computational Linguistics v.21 n.4 (2002) 543-565

21. Hirschman, L., Park, J. C., Tsujii, J., Wong, L. and Wu, C. H.: Accomplishments and challenges in literature data mining for biology. Bioinformatics Vol. 18 (2002) 1553-1561

Extracting Named Entities Using
Support Vector Machines

Yu-Chieh Wu[1], Teng-Kai Fan[1], Yue-Shi Lee[2], and Show-Jane Yen[2]

[1] Department of Computer Science and Information Engineering,
National Central University, No.300, Jhong-Da Rd.,
Jhongli City, Taoyuan County 32001, Taiwan, R.O.C
{bcbb, ceya}@db.csie.ncu.edu.tw
[2] Department of Computer Science and Information Engineering,
Ming Chuan University, No.5, De-Ming Rd, Gweishan District,
Taoyuan County 333, Taiwan, R.O.C
{leeys, sjyen}@mcu.edu.tw

Abstract. Identifying proper names, like gene names, DNAs, or proteins is useful to help researchers to mining the text information. Learning to extract proper names in natural language text is a named entity recognition (NER) task. Previous studies focus on combining abundant human made rules, trigger words, to enhance the system performance. However these methods require domain experts to build up these rules and word set which relies on lots of human efforts. In this paper, we present a robust named entity recognition system based on support vector machines (SVM). By integrating with rich feature set and the proposed mask method, the system performance is satisfactory on the MUC-7 and biology named entity recognition tasks which outperforms famous machine learning-based method, such as hidden markov model (HMM), and maximum entropy model (MEM). We compare our method to previous systems that were performed on the same data set. The experiments show that when training with the MUC-7 data set, our system achieves 86.4 in $F_{(\beta=1)}$ rate and 81.57 for the biology corpus. Besides, our named entity system is able to handle real time processing applications, the turn around time on a 63 K words document set is less than 30 seconds.

1   Introduction

Named entity (NE) is the structured information referring to predifined proper names, like persons, locations and organizations. Automatically Extracting proper names is useful to many problems such as machine translation, information retrieval, question answering and summarization. The goal of named entity recognition is to classify names into some particular categories from text. In biology text data, the named entity system can automatically extract the predefined names (like protein and DNA names) from raw documents.

The Message Understanding Conference (MUC) has provided the benchmark for named entity systems that performed a variety of information extraction tasks. In recent years, there have been other system development competitions which mainly focus on different language NER tasks (IREX, CoNLL-2002, 2003).

E.G. Bremer et al. (Eds.): KDLL 2006, LNBI 3886, pp. 91–103, 2006.
© Springer-Verlag Berlin Heidelberg 2006

NER is a fundamental task but it is the core of NLP system, therefore the performance of system will directly affect by this indispensable technology. Over the past decades, a considerable number of studies have been addressed on developing automatically named entity systems which can be categorized into three classes,

1. Rule-base NE system (Humphrey, 1998): This approach focus on extracting proper names using lots of human-made rule set. However, the rule-based NE systems lack of the ability of portability and robustness. The high cost of the rule maintain increases even though the data is slightly changed.
2. Machine Learning-based NE system (Bikel, 1999; Borthwick, 1998; Chieu, and Ng, 2002): To construct a machine learning-based NE system requires preparing labelled training data. Unlike the rule-based method, this approach can be easily port to different domain or languages.
3. Hybrid NE system (Mikheev et al., 1998; Borthwick, 1998): Using the combination of rule-based and machine learning-based approaches.

In recent years, many machine learning-based NE systems become more popular, and widely used in many applications, such as Hidden Markov Model (HMM) (Bikel et al., 1999), Maximum Entropy Model (MEM) (Borthwick, 1998), Decision Trees (Paliouras et al., 2000) and Support Vector Machines (SVM) (Takeuchi, and Collier, 2002). Especially, HMM-based approaches take only few seconds to train the examples. As for others, such as MEM, Decision trees and SVM, have flexible ability for modeling contextual information, and furthermore these approaches improves system performance.

Far from being considered a closed problem, several studies tried to enhance results on the NER task over past years. By encoding with eternal resources, e.g., part-of-speech taggers, human made lexicons, and create more training data (Mikheev et al., 1998), the high accuracy were obtained. Nevertheless the combinations of exteranl knowledges requires lots of human efforts. For example, Zhou and Su (Zhou and Su, 2002) propose reinforcement on original system by adding manually constructed trigger words. In developing an elaborated trigger word set is difficult for most cases. Since constructing these trigger words requires a domain experts and abundant thesaurus, like WordNet.

In this paper, we present a machine learning-based NE system by using SVMs. By integrating with rich feature set and the proposed mask method, high-performance result is obtained. Different from previous SVM-based NE systems, our method achieved higher performance and efficiency which is improved by working with linear kernel. For real time processing usage, our NE system can extract 2000 tokens per second. Our method is able to be port in different domain easily without re-writing rules or re-constructing trigger words. In the MUC-7 NE task, our method outperforms previous MEM-based method (Chieu, and Ng, 2002; Borthwick, 1998), and achieved the state-of-the-art performance on the biology corpus. In comparison to previous SVM-based and HMM-based NE systems (Takeuchi and Collier, 2001), our method is more robust in different NE tasks.

The rest of this paper is organized as follows. Section 2 introduces the fundamental of support vector machines. Section 3 explains our named entity model. The mask method will be described in Section 4. Experimental results are showed in Section 5. In Section 6, we draw the concluding remarks and future work.

2 Support Vector Machines

SVM are supervised machine learning algorithms for binary classification, which has been successfully applied to a number of particle problems (Kudoh and Matsumoto, 2001; Gimenez and Marquez, 2003). Let us define the training examples each of which labeled with either positive or negative class tag, as: $(x_1, y_1)...(x_n, y_n)$, where $x_i \in R^n$, y_i {+1, -1}, that x_i is a feature vector of the i_th example represented by and n-dimensional vector. y_i is the label of the i_{th} example. (either +1 for positive or -1 for negtive). N is the total number of training examples derived from the training set.

In basic form, a SVM learns to find a linear hyperlane that separate both positive and negative examples with maximal margin. This learning bias has proved to have good properties in terms of generalization bounds for the induced classifiers. Find the maximal margin can be express as follows:

$$(w. \ x) + b = 0, (w \in R^n, b \in R) \tag{1}$$

Suppose the hyperlane separate the training data into positive and negative parts, such that

$$y_i (w. \ x_i) \geqq 1 \tag{2}$$

However, several of such separating hyperlane exists (see Fig. 1 left hand side) SVM finds the optimal hyperlane that maximize the margins between the nearest examples to the hyperlane. The margin (M) and the lines can be expressed as:

$$w. \ x + b = \pm 1, M = 2 / \|w\| \tag{3}$$

To maximize this margin is equivalent to minimize the $\| w \|$. This is equivalent to solve the following optimization problem.

$$\text{Minimize: } (1/2) \|w\|^2 \tag{4}$$

$$\text{Subject to: } y_i [(w. \ x_i) + b] \geqq 1. \tag{5}$$

Examples which lied on the dashed lines are called support vectors. It is known that the optimal hyperlane can be obtained even if we remove all training examples except for the support vectors. Since SVM only solves the binary classification problem, we must extend it to multi-class classifiers to recognize named entities. Among

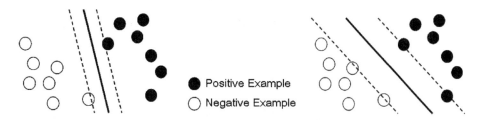

Fig. 1. A toy example of two possible separating hyperplanes

several multi-class SVMs, we employ the simple one-against-all method. In other words, SVM is trained for every Name Entity in order to distinguish between examples of this class and all the rest.

3   Named Entity Extraction Model

The named entity structure of a sentence can be encoded using IOB2 style (Tjong Kim Sang, 2000, 2002). The major constituents of the IOB2 style are B/I/O tags and the named entity class which represent the begin (B) of a named entity, the interior (I) of a named entity. When a word is assigned the tag "O", it does not a named entity word. For example, the sentence, "The adaptor protein Gads is a Grb2.". could be represented as,

The(O) adaptor(B-Protein) protein(I-Protein) Gads(I-Protein) is(O) a(O) Grb2(B-Protein) .(O)

As shown above, word "adaptor" indicates the beginning word of the named class Protein which is tagged as B-Protein, while the "protein", and "Gads" are encoded as I-Protein tag since they are the inside components of the named class. When the chunk structure is encoded as IOB-like style, a chunking problem can be viewed as a word-classification task, i.e., identify IOB chunk tag for each word. The optimal "class" of the current word is determined by encoding the context word features. Many common NLP components, for example Part-of-Speech (POS) taggers [7], and shallow parsers [17] [19] were presented according to the "word-classification" structure. The proposed named entity recognition model is also developed followed the same scheme. Fig. 2 illustrates the proposed model. Each component of our model is described bellow.

Pre-processing: At first, the input text strings should be segmented into tokens with a simple tokenizer.

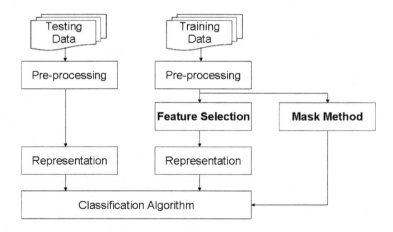

Fig. 2. System architecture of the proposed named entity system

Feature Selection: At this step, rich feature sets are selected to encode the information of each word (see Section 3.1).

Mask Method: The mask method produces more training instances for the classification algorithm, more detail descriptions can be found in Section 4.

Representation: This step is used to represent each training example to learn. According to the selected features, the whole training data can be encoded as a set of vectors.

Classification Algorithm: The classification algorithm automatically learns to classify testing data from the produced training examples at previous stage. Currently, there are many classification algorithms and we select one of the famous method to.

Other than the mask method, the other parts are well-known techniques. However, the selected features also influent on the system performance. Thus, we further introduce the two components in the following sections.

3.1 Feature Set

In general, the contextual information is often used as the seed feature; the other features can then be derived based on the surrounding words. In this paper, we adopt the following feature types.

- **Lexical information (Unigram)**
- **Affix (2~4 suffix and prefix letters)**
- **Previous NE information (UniChunk)**
- **Possible NE classes:** For the current word to be tagged, we recall its possible named entity tags in the training data and use its possible named class as a feature.

Table 1. Token feature category list

Feature description	Example text	Feature description	Example text
1-digit number	3	Number contains alpha and slash	1/10th
2-digit number	30	All capital word	NCU
4-digit number	2004	Capital period (only one)	M.
Year decade	2000s	Capital periods (more than one)	I.B.M.
Only digits	1234	Alpha contains money	US$
Number contains one slash	3/4	Alpha and periods	Mr.
Number contains two slash	2004/8/10	Capital word	Taiwan
Number contains money	$199	Number and alpha	F-16
Number contains percent	100%	Initial capitalization	Mr., Jason
Number contains hyphen	1-2	Inner capitalization	WordNet
Number contains comma	19,999	All lower case	am, is, are
Number contains period	3.141	Others	3∨4
Number contains colon	08:00		

Additionally, we also add more *N*-gram features, including **Bigram, and BiNE**. In addition, we design an orthographic feature type called **Token feature**, where each term will be assigned to a token class type via the pre-defined word category mapping. Table 1 lists the defined token feature types. Although this feature type is language dependent, many languages still contain Arabic numbers and symbols. Besides, many researches indicated that the use of gazetteers can help to find more named entity terms (Chieu and Ng, 2002; Zhou and Su, 2002). In this paper, we followed the same scheme to collect the person, location, and organization gazetteers from the web sites[1]. The feature Gazetteers is used when the word can not be found in the lexical information.

We employ SVM^{light} as the classification algorithm, which has been shown to perform well on classification problems (Joachims, 2001; Gimenez and Marquez, 2003). To take the time efficiency into account, we choose the linear kernel type. As discussed in many studies, the other kernels do not as efficient as the linear kernels (Gimenez and Marquez, 2003).

4 Mask Method

In real world, training data is insufficient, since only a subset of the vocabularies can appear in the testing data. During testing, if a term is an unknown word (or one of its context words is unknown), then the lexical related features, like unigram, and bigram are disabled, because the term information is not found in the training data. In this case, the name class of this word is mainly determined by the remaining features. Usually, this will low down the system performance.

The most common way for solving unknown word problem is to use different feature sets for unknown words and divide the training data into several parts to collect unknown word examples (Gimenez and Marquez, 2003). However, the selection of these feature sets for known word and unknown word were often arranged heuristically and it is difficult to select when the feature sets are different. Moreover, they just extract the unknown word examples and miss the instances that contain unknown contextual words.

To solve this problem, the mask method is designed to produce additional examples that contain "weak" lexical information to train. If the classification algorithm can learn these instances, in testing, it is able to classify the examples which contain insufficient lexical information. Fig. 3 summarizes the proposed mask algorithm. Suppose we have derived lexicon-related features from the training dataset, including unigram dictionary (UD), bigram dictionary (BD), and possible NE class dictionary (ID) from all training parts except for part i. We then generate new training examples by mapping the new dictionary set F_i (F_i is created from F by replacing UD, BD, and ID with UD_i, BD_i, and ID_i respectively). Technically, we create a mask m_i of length $|F|$ where a bit is set for a lexicon in F_i and clear if the lexicon is not in F_i. We then generate new vectors for all examples by logical "AND" it with mask m_i. Thus, items which appear only in part i are regarded as unknown words. The process is repeated for k times and a total of $(k+1)*n$ example vectors are generated (n is the original number of training words).

---

[1] Company names: http://www.yahoo.com, person names: http://www.babynames.com, location names: http://www.geohive.com/

Step 0. Let F be the feature dictionary constructed in Section 3.1. Let lexical-related unigram dictionary

UD: the unigram dictionary, BD: the bigram dictionary,

ID: the known label dictionary

$(UD \subseteq F, BD \subseteq F,$ and $ID \subseteq F)$

Step 1. Divide the training data into k ($k=2$) parts.

$$T = \bigcup_{i=1}^{k} T_i$$

Step 2. For each part i, mask T_i by compute $T' = T - T_i$

2.1 Generate lexical-related dictionaries from T'

UD_i: the unigram dictionary of T';

BD_i: the bigram dictionary of T';

ID_i: the known label dictionary of T'

F_i is created from F by replacing $UD/BD/ID$ with $UD_i/BD_i/ID_i$

2.2 Create a vector m_i of length $|F|$ where a bit is set for a lexicon in F_i and clear if the lexicon is not in F_i.

2.3 For each training example v_j represented by feature F,

$$v_j' = v_j \text{ AND } m_i$$

2.4 Output $S_i = \bigcup_{j=1}^{N} v_j'$

Step 3. Go to Step 1 until all parts has been processed

Fig. 3. The mask method algorithm

Let us illustrate a simple example. Assume that the unigram is the only one selected feature, and each training instance is represented via mapping to the unigram dictionary. At the first stage, the whole training data set generates the original unigram dictionary, T: $(A,B,...,G)$. After splitting the training data (Step 1), two disjoint sub-parts are produced. Assume step 2 to 2.1 produces two new unigram dictionaries, T_1: (B,C,D,E) by masking the first part, and T_2: (A,C,D,F,G) by masking the second part. Thus, the mask for the first partition is $(0,1,1,1,1,0,0)$ which reserves the common items in T and T_1. For a training example with features (A,C,F), the generated vectors is (C) since A and F are masked (Step 2.3). We use the same way to collect training examples from the second part.

The mask technique can transform the known lexical features into unknown lexical features and add k times training materials from the original training set. Thus, the original data can be reused effectively. As outlined in Fig. 3, new examples are generated through mapping into the masked feature dictionary set F_i. This is quite different from previous approaches, which employed variant feature sets for unknown words. The proposed method aims to emulate examples that do not contain lexical information, since named entity extraction errors often occur due to the lack of lexical features. Traditionally, the learners are given sufficient and complete lexical information; therefore, the trained models cannot generalize examples that contain incomplete lexical information. By including incomplete examples, the learners can take the effect of unknown words into consideration and adjust weights on lexical related features.

5 Experimental Results

In this section, we will report the experimental results of our system for both standard MUC-7 named entity, and a famous biology named extraction tasks. The MUC-7 data collection was derived from the articles of the air-accidents. The biology corpus was collected from 100 MEDLINE abstracts in the domain of molecular biology annotated for the nameds of genes and gene products (Tateishi et al., 2001; Takeuchi and Collier, 2002). Table 1 and 2 summaries the number of tokens for each named class of the MUC-7 and biology corpus.

For the MUC-7 data collections, the official released data consists of three parts, training, testing, and two dryrun data for development. Almost previous studies directly use the two dryrun data sets as a part of training set (Chieu and Ng, 2002). We follow the same settings and evaluates the system performance by estimates the accuracy on the testing data. On the other hand, there was not a standard testing set for the biology corpus. Thus, we evaluate our system by performing 10 cross-validation.

Table 2. Features of MUC-7 corpus

	# of tokens (Train)	# of tokens (Dryrun1)	# of tokens (Dryrun2)	# of tokens (Test)
DATE	1854	478	1811	2160
LOCATION	2134	437	2037	1559
MONEY	293	32	152	675
ORGANIZATION	3767	789	3549	3711
PERCENT	70	6	101	225
PERSON	2014	434	2101	1418
TIME	587	143	485	475
NOT-A-NAME	77346	17053	72503	53440
Total	**88065**	**19372**	**82739**	**63663**

Table 3. Features of biology corpus

	# of tokens	Descriptions
DNA	950	DNAs, DNA groups, regions and genes
PROTEIN	3230	Proteins, Protein groups, families, complexes and substructures
RNA	56	RNAs, RNA groups, regions and genes
SOURCE.cl	263	Cell line
SOURCE.ct	773	Cell type
SOURCE.mo	28	Mono-organism
SOURCE.mu	65	Multi-celled organism
SOURCE.sl	82	Sublocation
SOURCE.ti	60	Tissue
SOURCE.vi	140	Virus
Others	20477	Not-a-name

The performance of the named entity task is measured by three rates, recall, precision, and $F_{(\beta)}$. CoNLL released a perl-script evaluator[2] that enabled us to estimate the three rates automatically.

There are three parameters in our chunking system: the context window size, the frequent threshold for each feature dictionary, and the number of division parts for the unknown word examples (N). We set the first two parameters to 3, and 2 respectively as previous named entity systems (Takeuchi and Collier, 2002). Since the training time taken by SVMs scales exponentially with the number of input examples (Joachims, 2001), we set N as two for all of the following experiments.

5.1 Experimental Result

Our method is evaluated in the MUC-7 and biology dataset. Table 4 gives the overall named entity extraction results of each name class of the MUC-7 collections. The best system performance was obtained via integrating with the web-collected gazetteers. Without using the gazetteers, the performance is decreased to 77.45 in $F_{(\beta=1)}$ rate. Table 5 lists the comparisons of the previous top named entity system in the MUC-7 collections. Our method achieved the fourth best performance.

Table 4. System performance for MUC-7 collections in different named entity class

	Recall	Precision	$F_{(\beta=1)}$
DATE	88.24	73.02	79.91
LOCATION	90.97	92.21	91.59
MONEY	74.59	59.73	66.34
ORGANIZATION	88.52	82.65	85.49
PERCENT	88.24	90.00	89.11
PERSON	93.01	96.16	94.56
TIME	96.15	67.57	79.37
All	**89.57**	**83.46**	**86.40**

Table 5. Comparisons of named entity extraction performance for MUC-7 collections

	Size of training data	$F_{(\beta=1)}$
HMM chunk tagger	80,000 tokens	94.50
LTG system 98' (Mikheel et al., 1998)	Unknown	93.39
IdentiFinder 99' (Bikel et al., 1999)	790,000 tokens	90.44
Our method	**180,000 tokens**	**86.40**
MENERGI (Chieu and Ng, 2002)	180,000 tokens	85.22
MENE (Borthwick, 1998)	321,000 tokens	84.22

In another experiments, we directly port our named entity system to the biology corpus without any parameter tuning and model adjustment. Table 6 summarizes the overall performance in different name class for the biology corpus. As shown in Table 6, our method could recognize correctly most Protein names in text, but failure in the RNA, and Source.mo classes. It is worth to note that in the biology corpus, these

---

[2] http://lcg-www.uia.ac.be/conll2000/chunking/conlleval.txt

terms are not frequent while the protein words occupy 15% of the training set. Therefore to increase the training data of the other biology names is reasonably useful. In the biology named entity recognition task, we did not use the web-collected gazetteers since the improvement is marginal. The comparison of this task is listed in Table 7. In this task, our method obtained the best performance compared to previous studies (Takeuchi and Collier, 2002).

Table 6. System performance for biology corpus in different named entity class

	Precision	Recall	$F_{(\beta=1)}$
DNA	76.04	60.69	67.14
PROTEIN	82.39	87.81	**84.99**
RNA	56.66	30.99	38.13
SOURCE.cl	83.75	69.37	73.82
SOURCE.ct	81.30	86.41	83.66
SOURCE.mo	65.00	45.00	52.00
SOURCE.mu	85.31	73.71	75.79
SOURCE.sl	69.61	69.78	69.10
SOURCE.ti	71.29	52.03	56.37
SOURCE.vi	79.92	78.82	78.52
All	81.40	81.74	**81.57**

Table 7. Comparisons of named entity extraction performance for biology corpus

	Precision	Recall	$F_{(\beta=1)}$
Our method	**81.40**	**81.74**	**81.57**
SVM1 (Takeuchi and Collier, 2002)	75.89	68.09	71.78
HMM (Takeuchi and Collier, 2002)	73.10	58.95	70.97
SVM2 (Takeuchi and Collier, 2002)	--	--	65.63

Table 8 lists the improvement results of the mask method in the two named entity tasks. In these experiments, we focus on actual system performance in the unknown and known word recognition rate. As listed in Table 8, the mask method actually improves the system performance in terms of unknown word and known word parts. In the biology corpus, the mask method significantly enhances the recognition rate.

Table 8. The improvement by the mask method on the known and unknown words

	MUC-7	Biology Corpus
Unknown	81.34 → 83.27	68.25 → 69.50
Known	86.31 → 87.47	80.51 → 83.67
Total	85.13 → 86.40	78.82 → 81.57

5.2 Comparison

The MUC-7 collection is one of the most popular named entity benchmarking corpus. We compare our method with famous named entity systems that were performed on the same data set. Table 5 lists the relevant named entity system performance of the MUC-7 collection. It is clearly that the HMM chunk tagger achieved the best performance (94.50). In their studies, they made use of manually constructed trigger word set, proper name gazetteers. Note that the former components improves almost 12 in $F_{(\beta=1)}$ rate. It is unfairly to compare with most named entity systems, since most of them only made use of auto-collected gazetteers rather than human made trigger word set. The second best performance was obtained by LTG's named entity system (Mikheel et al., 1998). Their system was a hybrid method that combined with the machine learning approaches and human made rule set. They did not explicitly reveal the number of training size. The third best system is the BBN's IdentiFinder (Bikel et al., 1999) which made use of four times larger training set than the MUC-7 official released collections. To fairly compare with these systems is difficult because they employed various manually constructed rules, trigger words, larger training materials, and proper name gazetteers.

On the contrary, our method and the two maximum entropy-based systems (Chieu and Ng, 2002; Borthwick, 1998) only combined with an auto-collected gazetteer from the Internet. In terms of system portability and domain-dependency, the three named entity systems could be easily ported to different domain and languages. Even the lake of domain-specific gazetteers, the basic performance is reliable. For example, in the biology corpus, our method was directly ported without modifying the rules, trigger words.

On the other hand, our method outperforms the other named entity system in the biology corpus. Table 7 lists the related system performance of the biology corpus. In this comparison, we faily perform 10 cross-validation which was consistent with Takeuchi and Collier's work without using any gazetteers. In their studies, they also employed a Part-of-Speech (POS) tagger to obtain the syntactic features. They also demonstrated that their SVM-based named entity system (SVM+) outperformed the HMM-based. They best system performance of their results was reached by employed the polynomial kernel to SVM. Even the performance of their SVM slightly outperformed the HMM-based approach, the time cost is another problem. On the contrary, our method is not only simple but much more efficient than previous SVM-based system by working on the simple linear kernel SVM. In our close experiments, when our system combined with the polynomial kernel, both learning and testing time was largely increased (training: 25 minutes v.s. 8 hours, testing: 2000 tokens/sec v.s. 20 tokens/sec). For real time purpose, like document retrieval and question answering, such a slow named entity systems is difficult to use.

6 Conclusion

In this paper, we have presented a named entity system that allowed us to extract proper names in text. In particular we addressed on both general and biology named entity extraction problems. By using our method, the pre-defined named entities could be identified correctly without integrating human-made trigger words, or rules. By using the rich feature set and the proposed mask method, our method achieves reliable result on different named entity tasks. The experimental results show that our method achieves state-of-the-art performance in the biology named entity extraction (81.57), and reach 86.40 in F rate for the MUC-7 collections. The online demonstration of our named entity systems can be found at (http://140.115.155.87/bcbb/NER.htm).

References

1. Bikel, D., Schwartz, R., and Weischedel, R. An algorithm that learns what's in a name. Machine Learning (1999) 211-231.
2. Borthwick, A.: Maximum entropy approach to named entity recognition, PhD dissertation, 1998.
3. Brill, E.: Transformation-based error-driven learning and natural language processing: a case study in part of speech tagging. Computational Linguistics (1995) 21(4):543-565.
4. Carreras, X. and Marquez, L.: Phrase recognition by filtering and ranking with perceptrons. Proceedings of the International Conference on Recent Advances in Natural Language Processing (2003).
5. Chieu, H. L., and Ng, H. T.: Name entity recognition: a maximum entropy approach using global information, International Conference on Computational Linguistics (COLING) (2002) 190-196.
6. Giménez, J. and Márquez, L.: Fast and accurate Part-of-Speech tagging: the SVM approach revisited. In Proceedings of the International Conference on Recent Advances in Natural Language Processing (2003) 158-165.
7. Humphreys, K., Gaizauskas, R., Azzam, S., Huyck, C., Mitchell, B., Cunningham, H. and Wilks, Y.: University of Sheffield: Description of the. LaSIE-II System as Used for MUC-7. In Proceedings of 7th Message Understanding Conference (1998) 1-12.
8. Isozaki, H., and Kazawa, H.: Efficient support vector classifiers for named entity recognition. In Proceedings of the 17th Computational Linguistics (COLING) (2002) 390-396.
9. Joachims, T.: A statistical learning model of text classification with support vector machines. In Proceedings of the 24th ACM SIGIR Conference on Research and Development in Information Retrieval (2001) 128-136.
10. Kudoh, T. and Matsumoto, Y.: Chunking with support vector machines. In Proceedings of the 2nd Meetings of the North American Chapter and the Association for the Computational Linguistics (2001).
11. Paliouras, G., Karkaletsis, V., Petasis, G., and Spyropoulos, C. D.: Learning decision trees for named-entity recognition and classification. In Proceedings of the 14th European Conference on Artificial Intelligence (ECAI) (2000).
12. Mayfield, J., McNamee, P., and, Piatko, C.: Named entity recognition using hundreds of thousands of features. In Proceedings of the 7th Conference on Natural Language Learning (CoNLL) (2003) 184-187.
13. McNamee, P., and Mayfield, J.: Entity Extraction without Language-Specific Resources. In Proceedings of the 6th Conferrence on Natural Language Learning (CoNLL) (2002) 183-186.
14. Mikheev, A., Grover, C., and Moens, M.: Description of the LTG system used for MUC-7. Proceedings of 7th Message Understanding Conference (1998) 1-12.
15. Mikheev, A., Moens, M. and Grover, C.: Named entity recognition without gazetteers. In Proceedings of the 37th Annual Meeting of the Association for Computational Linguistics (ACL) (1999) 1-8.

16. Takeuchi, K. and Collier, N.: Use of support vector machines in extended named entity recognition. In Proceedings of the 6th Conference on Natural Language Learning (CoNLL) (2002) 119-125.
17. Tjong Kim Sang , E. F. and Buchholz, S.: Introduction to the CoNLL-2000 shared task: chunking. In Proceedings of Conference on Natural Language Learning (CoNLL) (2000) 127-132.
18. Tjong Kim Sang, E. F., and Fien, D. M.: Introduction to the CoNLL-2003 Shared Task: Language-Independent Named Entity Recognition. In Proceedings of the 7th Conference on Natural Language Learning (CoNLL) (2003) 142-147.
19. Zhou, G. D., and Su, J.: Name entity recognition using an HMM-based chunk tagger. In Proceedings of the 40th Annual Meeting of the Association for Computational Linguistics (ACL) (2002) 473-480.

Extracting Initial and Reliable Negative Documents to Enhance Classification Performance

Hui Wang and Wanli Zuo

College of Computer Science and Technology, Jilin University, Key Laboratory of
Symbolic Computation and Knowledge Engineering of the Ministry of Education,
Changchun 130012, China
durational@163.com

Abstract. Most existing text classification work assumes that training data are
completely labeled. In real life, some information retrieval problems can only
be described as learning a binary classifier from a set of incompletely labeled
examples, where a small set of labeled positive examples and a very large set of
unlabeled ones are provided. In this case, all of the traditional text classification
methods can't work properly. In this paper, we propose a method called
Weighted Voting Classifier, which is an improved 1-DNF algorithm. Experimental results on the Reuters-21578 set show that our algorithm Weighting
Voting Classifier outperforms PEBL and one-class SVM in terms of F measure.
Weighting Voting Classifier can achieve high F score when comparing with
PEBL and one-class SVM. Furthermore, the reduction of iterations is 2.26
when comparing the method of PEBL with ours.

1 Introduction

Automatic text categorization or classification is the process of assigning predefined
category labels to new documents based on the classifier learnt from training examples. In traditional classification, training data are labeled with the same set of
pre-defined categories or class labels and labeling is often done manually. It is often
tedious and expensive to hand-label large amount of training data. In some environment, we must train our staff to label documents properly, such as in the library. Thus
recently, semi-supervised learning algorithms have been defined from a small set of
labeled data with the help of unlabeled data. Such approaches include using Expecta-
tion Maximization to estimate maximum posteriori parameters [1], [2], and using
transductive inference for support vector machines [3].

In many practical classification applications such as web pages analysis, labeled data
can be short of supply but unlabeled data are more readily available. Many proposed
algorithms can exploit the unlabeled data to improve performance on the classification
task. One class of algorithms is based on a two-step strategy. These algorithms include
S-EM [4], PEBL [5], and Roc-SVM [6]. Bing Liu [7] perform a comprehensive evaluation of all possible combinations of the methods which were used in the two steps and
propose a new approach to solve the classification problem based on a biased formulation of SVM, which was shown to be more accurate than existing techniques.

E.G. Bremer et al. (Eds.): KDLL 2006, LNBI 3886, pp. 104–111, 2006.
© Springer-Verlag Berlin Heidelberg 2006

In this paper, we propose a new method, an improved 1-DNF algorithm which was proposed in PEBL previously, to employ the unlabeled data for improving the performance of text classification task. This paper is organized as follows. In the next section, we will overview some related works in this domain. In section 3, we will discuss our proposed technique. The actual implementation and experimental results are discussed in section 4. In the end, the conclusions and future works are discussed in section 5.

2   Related Works

A theoretical study of Probably Approximately Correct (PAC) learning from positive and unlabeled examples was done in [8]. Since then, some experimental attempts have been tried using k-DNF of decision trees to learn from positive and unlabeled data [9], [10]. Sample complexity results from learning by maximizing a number of unlabeled examples labeled as negative while constraining the classifier to label all the positive examples correctly were presented in [4]. Traditional text classification techniques require labeled training examples of all classes to build a classifier [11]. They are thus not suitable for building classifiers using only positive and unlabeled examples.

The techniques of S-EM, PEBL and Roc-SVM were reported in [4], [5], [6] respectively. Unlike these techniques which are based on the two-step strategy, Lee, W [12] design a logistic regression technique to solve the problem. It is also possible to discard the unlabeled data and learn only from the positive data. This is done in the one-class SVM [13], [14], which try to learn the support from the distribution of positive examples only. Our experimental results show that its performance is rather poorer than other learning methods (see Section 4).

In the end, our work is related to using a small labeled data set and a large unlabeled data set [15], [16], [17], [18], [19]. In all these works, a small set of labeled examples of each class and a large unlabeled data set are used to train classifiers. Experimental results show that the unlabeled data can help the process of learning a classifier. Without these unlabeled data, classifier can not achieve high precision of classification.

3   The Proposed Technique

In this section, we present our proposed method, which also consists of two steps: (1) extracting some reliable negative documents from the unlabeled data set, (2) applying SVM iteratively to build a classifier. In the following part, we interpret these two steps in turn according to [7].

3.1   Step 1: Finding Reliable Negative Documents

The 1-DNF method (see Figure 1) in PEBL [5] first builds a positive feature set PF which contains words that occur in the positive data set P more frequently than in the unlabeled data set U (lines 1-5). In lines 6-9, it tries to filter out possible positive documents from U. A document which does not have any positive features PF is regarded as a reliable negative document.

1. Assume the word feature set
   be $\{x_1, x_2, \cdots, x_n\}$, $x_i \in U \cup P$
2. Let positive feature set $PF = null$
3. for $i = 1$ to n
4.   if ($freq(x_i, P)/|P| > freq(x_i, U)/|U|$) then
5. $PF = PF \cup \{x_i\}$
6. $RN = U$
7. for each document $d \in U$
8.   if $\exists x_j freq(x_j, d) > 0$ and $x_j \in PF$ then
9. $RN = RN - \{d\}$

Fig. 1. The 1-DNF method in PEBL

Obviously, there is one shortcoming in this technique: this algorithm only considers those features which occur more frequently in P than in U, but it does not take care of their absolute frequencies respectively. Thinking in this: if a feature has 1% frequencies in P and 0.5% frequencies in U, then what can we do. We have to put it into PF set according to 1-DNF algorithm. This may be a wrong decision, especially when we have only a small number of positive documents. In order to deal with above problem and enhance the performance of classification, we propose an improved 1-DNF algorithm (see Figure 2).

1. Assume the word feature set
   be $\{x_1, \cdots, x_n\}$, $x_i \in U \cup P$
2. Let positive feature set $PF = null$
3. Let negative feature set $NF = null$
4. for $i = 1$ to n
5.   if ($freq(x_i, P)/|P| > freq(x_i, U)/|U|$ and
           $freq(x_i, P)/|P| >= \lambda\%$)
6. $PF = PF \cup \{x_i\}$
7.   if ($freq(x_i, U)/|U| > freq(x_i, P)/|P|$ and
           $freq(x_i, U)/|U| >= \gamma\%$)
8. $NF = NF \cup \{x_i\}$
9. $RN_0 = null$
10. for each document $d \in U$
11.   if ($\forall x_i \in PF$ and $freq(x_i, d) == 0$ or
           $\sum_{x_j \in d, x_j \in NF} x_j >= \sum_{x_i \in d, x_i \in PF} x_i + m$) then
12. $RN_0 = RN_0 \cup \{d\}$

Fig. 2. The improved 1-DNF technique in Weighted Voting Classifier

Our method first builds a Positive Feature set PF which contains words that must satisfy the following two constraints: firstly, they must occur in the positive data set P more frequently than in the unlabeled data set U; secondly, their absolute frequencies in P larger than or equal λ percent (see lines 5-6). Unlike to PEBL, our method also builds up a Negative Feature set NF corresponding to PF (see lines 7-8). In lines 9-12, it tries to obtain initial Reliable Negative data set RN_0 from U. For each document which belongs to U, we can put it into Reliable Negative data set RN_0 data set if it satisfies one of the following two constraints: first, it does not contain any Positive Feature PF; second, it contains less Positive Feature PF than Negative Feature NF(see line 11). In our experiments, m is an integer and we let λ equal γ for simplicity. As for λ, we range it from 10 to 70 with interval of 10 to create a wide range of scenarios.

Noticing that: in PEBL, it may obtain a large amount of Reliable Negative Documents from U (see lines 6-9, in Fig. 1). To obtaining Reliable Negative Documents, it begins from $RN = U$ and then filters out all possible positive documents from U. As for Support Vector Machines (SVM, see next section 3.2), this may be a bad news in most cases. On the contrary to this, we begin with $RN_0 = null$ and then put reliable negative documents into RN_0 incrementally (see lines 9-12, in Fig. 2). We should do some experiments to verify our statements, but we do not at present and we think we could do.

3.2 Step 2: Training Classifier Using *SVM* [7]

Support Vector Machines (SVM) show that they can yield good generalization performance on a wide variety of classification problems, most recently on text categorization. The SVM integrates dimension reduction and classification. Its form looks like this: $f(x) = w^T x + b$, where $w^T x$ is the inner product between the weight vector w and the input vector x. SVM is used as a classifier by setting the class to 1 if $f(x) > 0$ and to -1 otherwise. The main idea of SVM is to select a hyperplane that separates the positive from negative examples while maximizing the smallest margin. Let a set of training examples be $\{(x_1, y_1), (x_2, y_2), \cdots, (x_n, y_n)\}$, where x_i is an input vector and y_i is its class label, $y_i \in \{1, -1\}$. The problem of finding the hyperplane can be stated as the following optimization problem:

$$\text{Minimize: } \frac{1}{2} w^T w$$
$$\text{Subject to: } y_i(w^T x_i + b) \geq 1, \quad i = 1, 2, \cdots, n .$$

To deal with cases where there may be no separating hyperplane due to noisy labels of both positive and negative training examples, the soft margin SVM is proposed [20], which is formulated as:

$$\text{Minimize: } \frac{1}{2} w^T w + C \sum_{i=1}^{n} \xi_i$$
$$\text{Subject to: } y_i(w^T x_i + b) \geq 1 - \xi_i, \quad i = 1, 2, \cdots, n ,$$

where $C \geq 0$ is a parameter that controls the amount of training errors allowed.

We adopt the same process which was used in PEBL (iterative SVM in PEBL) [5]. Unlike the technique of PEBL, we also decide which classifiers to use after SVM convergence. Because each iteration builds a different SVM classifier and also because SVM is sensitive to noise, if some iterations of SVM extract too many positive documents from U and put them into RN_0, the last SVM classifier may not be the best classifier. According to this, we propose a new method (see Figure 3) to decide what our final classifier looks like whereas in PEBL the last classifier is the result.

```
1.   PP = 10%P , P = P - PP , totalAccuracy = 0
2.   SVM₀ = SVM(RN₀, P)
3.   i = 0
4.   Loop
5.       accuracyᵢ stands for the precision
             when SVMᵢ applying to PP data set
6.       totalAccuracy+ = accuracyᵢ
7.       RN_{i+1} = SVMᵢ · classify(U)
8.       if RN_{i+1} = { } then Exit-Loop
9.       RN₀ = RN₀ ∪ RN_{i+1}
10.      U = U - RN_{i+1}
11.      i = i + 1
12.      SVMᵢ = SVM(RN₀, P)
13.  End Loop
```

$$14.\quad finalSVM = \sum_{i=0}^{n} \frac{accuracy_i}{totalAccuracy} SVM_i$$

Fig. 3. Algorithm for obtaining the final classifier

In our experiments, we reserve 10 percent of positive documents for calculating the precision of each SVM classifier (see line 1). In line 2, our algorithm first uses initial and reliable negative data set RN_0 obtained in Figure 2 and positive data set P to train a SVM classifier. In lines 4-13, iterations begin. For each obtained SVM classifiers, we calculate its precision and add its precision into total precision, which was noted by $totalAccuracy$ (see lines 5-6). Then, we use the classifier to go on deriving reliable negative documents from U (see line 7). Not getting any reliable negative documents, we exit our algorithm (see line 8). Otherwise, we put the derived reliable negative documents into RN_0 and subtract them from U also (see lines 9-10). Once again, we train another SVM classifier using new reliable negative documents RN_0 and positive data set P (see line 12). In line 14, we integrate all of these classifiers to obtain the final classifier- $finalSVM$. We name it the Weighted Voting Classifier (WVC) for our $finalSVM$ classifier, because we get it according to each classifier's precision. The higher precision a classifier is, the larger weight it gets.

4   Experimental Results

This section evaluates the proposed technique using the Reuters-21578 text collection, which is commonly used in evaluating text classification methods. The Reuters-21578 collection contains 21578 text documents. We used only the most populous 10 out of the135 topic categories. In our experiments, each category is used as the positive class, and the rest of the categories as the negative class. This gives us 10 datasets. We will compare our proposed algorithm with the method of PEBL and one-class SVM.

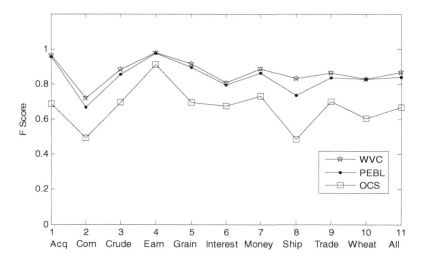

Fig. 4. F score of *PEBL*, *OCS* and Weighted Voting Classifier (*WVC*) on Reuters collection

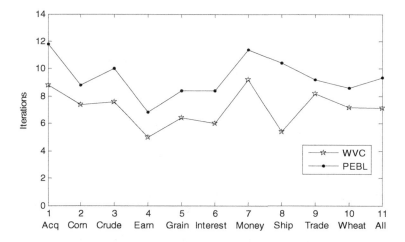

Fig. 5. Iterations of *PEBL* and Weighted Voting Classifier (*WVC*)on Reuters collection

For each data set, 30 percent of the documents (including both positive and unlabeled documents) are randomly selected as test documents, and the remaining is used to create training data sets. For each experiment in every data set, we randomly select q percent of documents from the positive class and put them into negative documents to get an unlabeled data set U. The remaining of 1-q percent positive documents are used as positive data set P. We range q from 10 percent to50 percent with interval of 10 for creating a wide range of scenarios.

For evaluating the performance of a text classifier, we employ the commonly used F score as one of our performance measures $F = 2pr/(p + r)$ (see Figure 4.), where p is the precision and r is the recall. We also compare our proposed algorithm with PEBL concerning iterations (see Figure 5.).

OCS stands for one-class SVM and WVC stands for our proposed Weighted Voting Classifier. From Figure 4, we can observe that our proposed technique outperforms the other two methods in terms of F values on, especially when comparing with one-class SVM. In our experiments, we find that we can obtain excellent performance when $\lambda = 10$ and $m = 3$. Based upon the results in Figure 4 and 5, we can draw two following conclusions:

- The performance of our technique is quite good when $\lambda = 10$ and m=3. It can achieve F score 0.8675 on average over ten categories, higher than PEBL 0.8401 and one-class SVM 0.6676.
- Furthermore, the reduction of iterations is 2.26 when comparing the method of PEBL with Weighted Voting Classifier.

Our proposed technique can identify quite a few initial reliable negative documents (see Figure 2) from the unlabeled data set U. With these reliable data sets, our SVM classifier converges fast and correctly.

5   Conclusions and Future Work

In this paper, we studied the problem of text classification using only partial information, i.e., using one class of labeled documents and a set of unlabeled ones. We propose an effective algorithm Weighted Voting Classifier to solve the problem. Weighted Voting Classifier first utilizes an improved 1-DNF algorithm to extract a set of initial reliable negative documents from the unlabeled data set, and then builds a set of SVM classifiers iteratively. Finally, we get final classifier according to each classifier's precision using weighted voting method. Experimental results show that our proposed technique is more efficient than one-class SVM and PEBL.

In the near future, we will remove the limitation $\lambda = \gamma$ and let λ and γ take different values if necessary. We also plan to do some experiments to compare our algorithm Weighted Voting Classifier with PEBL and one-class SVM on other data set, for example 20_newsgroups. At present, we only compare our algorithm Weighted Voting Classifier with PEBL and one-class SVM under the constraints of $m = 1,2,3$ on Reuters-21578 text collection, and leave it for our future work concerning m taking other integers.

Acknowledgements

This work is sponsored by the Natural Science Foundation of China under grant number 60373099.

References

1. Nigam, K., Ghani, R.: Analyzing the Applicability and Effectiveness of Co-training. Proceedings of CIKM-00, Ninth International Conference on Information and Knowledge Management (2000)86-93
2. M.-R, A., P, G.: Semi-supervised Learning with Explicit Misclassification Modeling. Proceedings of the 18th International Joint Conference on Artificial Intelligence (2003)
3. Joachims, T.: Transductive Inference for Text Classification Using Support Vector Machines. Proceedings of ICML-99, 16th International Conference on Machine Learning (1999) 200-209
4. Liu, B., Lee, W. S., Yu, P., Li, X.: Partially Supervised Classification of Text Documents. ICML-02
5. Yu, H., Han, J., Chang, K.: PEBL: Positive Example Based Learning for Web Page Classification Using SVM. KDD-02
6. Li, X., Liu, B.: Learning to Classify Text Using Positive and Unlabeled Data. IJCAI-03
7. Bing Liu, Yang Dai, Xiaoli Li, Wee Sun Lee, Philip, S. Yu.: Building Text Classifiers Using Positive and Unlabeled Examples. Proceedings of the Third IEEE International Conference on Data Mining (ICDM), (2003)179-187
8. Denis, F.: PAC Learning from Positive Statistical Queries. Proc. 9th International Conference on Algorithmic Learning Theory-ALT'987 (1998)112-126
9. Cortes, C., Vapnik, V.: Support Vector Networks. Machine Learning, 20 (1995) 273-297
10. Mase, H.: Experiments on Automatic Web Page Categorization for Ir System. Technical Report, Stanford University, http://citeseer.nj.nec.com/164846.html, (1998)
11. Yang, Y. and Liu, X.: A Re-examination of Text Categorization Methods. SIGIR-99
12. Lee, W. S., Liu, B.: Learning with Positive and Unlabeled Examples Using Weighted Logistic Regression. ICML-2003
13. Scholkopf, S., Platt, J., Shawe, J., Smola, A., Williamson, R.: Estimating the Support of a High-dimensional Distribution. Technical Report MSR-TR-99-87, Microsoft Research (1999)
14. Manevitz, L., Yousef, M.: One-class SVMs for Document Classification. J. of Machine Learning Research, 2 (2001)
15. Blum, A., Mitchell, T.: Combining Labeled and Unlabeled Data with Co-training. COLT-98
16. Ghani, R.: Combining Labeled and Unlabeled Data for Multiclass Text Categorization. ICML-(2002)
17. Goldman, S., Zhou, Y.: Enhancing Supervised Learning with Unlabeled Data. ICML-00 (2000)
18. Basu, S., Banerjee, A., Mooney, R.: Semi-supervised Clustering by Seeding. ICML-02 (2002)
19. Bennett, K., and Demiriz.: A Semi-supervised Support Vector Machines. Advances in Neural information processing systems 11 (1998)
20. Guyon, I., Boser, B., Vapnik, V.: Automatic Capacity Tuning of Very Large VC-dimension Classifiers. Advances in Neural Information Processing Systems, Vol. 5 (1993)

Detecting Invalid Dictionary Entries for Biomedical Text Mining

Hironori Takeuchi[1], Issei Yoshida[1], Yohei Ikawa[1],
Kazuo Iida[2], and Yoko Fukui[2]

[1] IBM Research, Tokyo Research Laboratory, IBM Japan, Ltd.,
Shimotsuruma 1623-14 Yamato-shi Kanagawa, Japan
[2] Research Institute of Bio-system Informatics, Tohoku Chemical Co., Ltd.,
Odouri 3-3-10 Morioka-shi Iwate, Japan

Abstract. In text mining, to calculate precise keyword frequency distributions in a particular document collection, we need to map different keywords that denote the same entity to a canonical form. In the life science domain, we can construct a large dictionary that contains the canonical forms and their variants based on the information from external resources and use this dictionary for the term aggregation. However, in this automatically generated dictionary, there are many invalid entries that have negative effects on the calculations of keyword frequencies. In this paper, we propose and test methods to detect invalid entries in the dictionary.

1 Introduction

Large amounts of information are stored and distributed as text and the amount of accessible textual data has been increasing rapidly. To extract knowledge and estimate trends in text data collections, text mining technologies are being developed and applied in some business areas [6]. In the life science area, there is a database called MEDLINE that contains over 14 million citations (abstracts) of biomedical articles going back to the 1960s. We can access this database by using PubMed. Many text mining technologies for information extraction and trend estimation using MEDLINE have been developed [9][12].

Text mining systems usually consist of two main components: a preprocessing information extraction component and a runtime component. In the preprocessing stage, we extract information from the text using Natural Language Processing (NLP), and the runtime component, by using this preprocessed data, calculates the distribution of the keywords' frequencies in the selected document collection and uses that information for the trend analysis. In the preprocessing stage, we want to aggregate synonymous expressions and spelling variations because there can be multiple expressions that are synonymous with a particular technical term in the life science domain. These multiple expression arise from synonyms or jargon with different spellings as well as from abbreviations or acronyms that can be derived from the canonical form [8]. If these expressions

E.G. Bremer et al. (Eds.): KDLL 2006, LNBI 3886, pp. 112–122, 2006.

are treated as different entities, we cannot accurately calculate the keyword frequencies. We also need to assign categories to particular keywords in the text. One of the most convenient methods for the term aggregation is to use a dictionary. The dictionary contains pairs consisting of a canonical form and a list of variants related to the canonical form, and also has the information about the categories that the canonical form belongs to. Variants include the synonymous expressions and spelling variations. At the NLP in the preprocessing stage, we reduce the variants in the text to their canonical form by using the dictionary.

For this term aggregation based on the dictionary search, we need to construct a dictionary that contains each technical term in a category and its variants. Though it takes a long time to construct such a large dictionary from scratch for the technical terms in the life science domain, we can use external databases as sources of the dictionary entries. There are databases that include biomedical information such as genes and proteins. From each record in such a database, we can extract its heading as the canonical form and other information for the entry's naming such as the variants for the canonical form. Usually, we collect dictionary information for each category such as a gene or a chemical compound from the corresponding external resources and integrate the information into a large dictionary [5]. In the life science text mining we use such an automatically constructed dictionary the term aggregation and category assignment.

However, there are many invalid entries that have negative impacts on the calculations of the keyword frequencies when using such an automatically constructed dictionary. Because external databases were not developed with text mining in mind and are not intended to be a lexical resources, deriving a dictionary from them has some problems. For example, many unrelated keywords including common nouns are registered as variants in the dictionary. If we use a dictionary that contains such entries, all of the occurrences of these common nouns will be replaced by the corresponding canonical form in the dictionary. As a result, we may calculate a meaningless distribution of the keyword frequencies and be led to false conclusions and nonexistent trends. To address this problem, it was proposed to detect common nouns registered as variants of the technical terms by using a lexical database for general English such as WordNet [3][11]. However, some of the invalid dictionary entries are not general English words and whether a dictionary entry is valid or invalid often depends on the purpose of the analysis in the life science area. Because the number of dictionary entries is very large, it is very difficult for us to examine whether each entry is valid for the purposes of a specific analysis. Therefore, if there were a list of dictionary entries that were judged to be invalid along with their invalidity scores, by using this list, we could easily improve the dictionary and customize it for our own purpose.

In this paper, we present the methods to detect invalid entries in the dictionary with scores that represent their invalidity and examine the effectiveness the new methods. The rest of this paper is organized as follows. In Section 2, we describe the dictionary used in text mining for biomedical documents and the invalid dictionary entries. In Section 3, we present our methods to detect invalid dictionary entries. In Section 4, we describe the outline of our system and the experiments, and cover the results in Section 5. Finally, we will discuss the results and offer conclusions regarding our proposed method.

2   Dictionary for Text Mining of Biomedical Documents

In this section, we describe the automatically generated dictionary used in our biomedical text mining and the negative aspects of this dictionary.

2.1   Dictionary Based on the External Resources

In the life science domain, the information acquired in experiments are registered in a database and electronically published via network. For example in Entrez Gene (previously called LocusLink [7]), there is extensive information, including the gene sequences. In this database, an "Official Symbol" is assigned to each gene as a headword and "Gene Aliases" and "Other Aliases" are assigned as aliases. From this information, we can extract an Official Symbol as the canonical form for the gene and the Gene Aliases and the Other Aliases as the variants corresponding to the canonical form and thus define dictionary entries for the gene category. There is a similar database for proteins (e.g. SwissProt[1]). In UMLS [2], technical terms in the life science domain are registered.

Using these external resources, for each category such as "genes", we can gather the dictionary entries that are defined as the pair of the canonical form and their variants. After integrating these dictionary information, we construct a huge dictionary and apply it for the term aggregation. For example, BioThe-saurus [5] consists of over 2.0 million dictionary entries extracted from multiple online resources. In the life science area, there are many technical terms and new terms are generated continually. In such a situation, it is very difficult to construct the dictionary from scratch by experts. So, this automatically generated dictionary is very useful for the term aggregation and the category assignment in the text mining.

2.2   Invalid Dictionary Entries and Their Negative Impact

Though this automatically generated dictionary is very useful, it often happens that the dictionary is contaminated with invalid entries because databases like Entrez Gene and SwissProt are not intended to be a lexical resources. One kind of contaminating entries is a common noun as the variant of a technical term. For example, when we search for the gene Spna2 (Gene ID:20740), we find that "brain" is registered in Other Aliases (July, 2005), so in the automatically generated dictionary, "brain" is one of the variants for the canonical form Spna2. If we leave this entry in the dictionary, all "brain" appeared in the text are recognized as Spna2 in the term aggregation process and the frequency of keyword "Spna2" will be very large. As the result, we may reach incorrect conclusions and see a non-existent trend related to Spna2. In addition to common nouns, there are many contaminant entries. For example, "EPO" is one of the Other

Table 1. Examples of the Invalid and Valid Dictionary Entries

canonical form	invalid variants	valid variants
IRF6	LPS, PPS	interferon regulatory factor 6
LEP	obesity, obese, ob, OB, LH	leptin precursor
PAX1	wt, un, hbs	Pax-1, HUP48
TNFRSR6	lpr, lymphoproliferation, APT1, Kis	APO-1, Fas

Aliases of the Official Symbol "TIMP1" in Entrez Gene, suggesting EPO is a variant of TIMP1. However, biology experts evaluated this entry and decided it was not suitable as a dictionary entry for the term aggregation and should be omitted from the dictionary. Whether variants that are not common nouns are not suitable sometimes depends on the purpose of the specific analysis. Table 1 shows other examples of the invalid and valid dictionary entries.

A method to delete invalid common nouns from the dictionary has been proposed [3][11]. In this method, common nouns that are registered as the variants of technical terms will be detected by using an electronic dictionary for general English words such as WordNet. However, as we mentioned above, some contaminating entries are not general English words and such entries cannot be detected by this method. In the next section, we define the invalid dictionary entries that interfere with the text mining of biomedical documents and propose methods to detect those invalid entries in the automatically generated dictionary.

3   Invalid Dictionary Entries Detection

In this section, we first define the invalid entries that should be excluded from the dictionary for the text mining. After that we present invalid entry detection methods that are based on comparison of the frequency distributions of the dictionary entries and the paraphrase expressions found for the canonical forms and their variants.

3.1   Definition of Invalid Dictionary Entry

Here we define an invalid dictionary entry for text mining. The goal of our work described here is to remove the dictionary entries that have negative impacts on the calculations of the keyword frequencies. Therefore we are not really concerned with every possibly invalid variants but only with the incorrect variants that adversely affect the analysis of a target document collection. In this paper, we consider not only the representation of the keyword but also its frequency in the document collection and define a risk score that shows the magnitude of negative impact on the calculation of the keyword frequencies if that specific keyword in the dictionary is invalid. By such a risk score, we can regard only keywords that are incorrect and have high frequencies as the invalid dictionary entries.

We denote f_s to be the frequency of a variant S in the test collection and ν to be the evaluation of the representation of the keyword by experts. ν is normalized over $[0, 1]$ (0:valid, 1:invalid). We define the risk score for S, $rs(S)$ as follows.

$$rs(S) = \left(\frac{\log(f_S + 1)}{\log(f_{max} + 1)} \cdot \nu \right)^a \tag{1}$$

where f_{max} is the maximum frequency of keywords in the test collection and a is the parameter for the slope of the risk function. By this definition, only keywords that are not suitable and have high frequencies have high risk values. We used the size of test collection for f_{max} and set $a = 0.5$ in the experiment. In our paper, we define S such that $rs(S) \geq 0.4$ to be an invalid dictionary entry.

3.2   Detection Using Frequency Information

It sometimes happens that a frequent keyword containing a common noun is assigned as the variant to a technical word that does not appear frequently in the text. Though we would regard a frequent variant to be invalid, whether or not the variant is a frequent term depends on the frequency of its canonical form. Therefore we consider the appearance probabilities of a variant and its canonical form and compare them for the evaluation of the dictionary entry. Let N be the size of the documents in the corpus, f_{c_i} be the frequency of a canonical form c_i, and f_{s_j} be the frequency of a variant s_j. From these values, we can estimate the respective appearance probabilities such that $p_{c_i} = \frac{f_{c_i}}{N}$ and $p_{s_j} = \frac{f_{s_j}}{N}$. Using these estimated values, we can calculate the Kullback-Leibler distance (KL distance) for the distribution of s_j relative to that of c_i as

$$KL(p_{s_j}, p_{c_i}) = p_{s_j} \log \frac{p_{s_j}}{p_{c_i}} + (1 - p_{s_j}) \log \frac{(1 - p_{s_j})}{(1 - p_{c_i})}. \tag{2}$$

We evaluate each dictionary entry consisting of the pair of a variant and its canonical form based on this KL distance. When the KL distance of a dictionary entry is over the threshold τ, we regard it as invalid and calculate $\hat{\nu}$, the estimation of ν for this entry such that $\hat{\nu} = 1$ (otherwise $\hat{\nu} = 0$). Here, τ is estimated by using the learning data that is described in Section 4.2.

3.3   Detection Using Paraphrase Expressions in the Documents

In the evaluation based on the comparisons between the occurrence probabilities, we regard the dictionary entry to be valid when the frequencies are the same as each other. In such a case, we leave the possibly erroneous entries in the dictionary. In other case, sometimes there is a variant that is much more commonly used by the researchers than its canonical form and which therefore appears frequently in the text. In this case, we regard such a dictionary entry to be invalid and remove it from the dictionary in spite of the valid entry, because the appearance probabilities of the variant is much larger than that of the canonical form. As a result, we lose useful information for the calculation of the canonical form's frequency. The evaluation using only the KL distance is not sufficient and we therefore need to reevaluate the evaluation results based on the KL distance.

For the reevaluation, we use the paraphrase expressions in the documents as evidence for the validity. We consider the retrieved documents that contain a variant and its canonical form. If the pair consisting of a variant and a canonical form is valid as a dictionary entry, it is expected that we will very likely find the paraphrase expressions such as "... *canonical (variant)* ..." in the retrieved documents. Therefore we define eight patterns for paraphrase expressions as follows:

$$p_1: \text{canonical (variant)} \quad p_2: \text{variant (canonical)}$$
$$p_3: \text{canonical/variant} \quad p_4: \text{variant/canonical}$$
$$p_5: \text{canonical : variant} \quad p_6: \text{variant : canonical}$$
$$p_7: \text{canonical - variant} \quad p_8: \text{variant - canonical.}$$

Using these patterns, we can investigate whether there are paraphrase expressions in the retrieved documents and reevaluate the results of the KL-distance-based evaluation. For each of the invalid and valid entries as detected by the KL-distance-based evaluation, we re-estimate $\hat{\nu}$ as

$$\hat{\nu} = \begin{cases} \alpha S_t(p_1)(1 - S_t(p_2)) + (1 - S_t(p_1)) \\ \quad \text{(reevaluation of invalid entries)} \\ \beta(1 - St(p_1 \text{ or } p_2 \text{ or } \cdots \text{ or } p_8)) \\ \quad \text{(reevaluation of valid entries)} \end{cases} \quad (3)$$

where $S_t(p)$ is a step function such that $S_t(p) = 1$ if p is contained in the retrieved documents. In the revaluation of an invalid entry, ν is estimated as $\hat{\nu} = 0$ if both p_1 and p_2 are found in the documents, is estimated as $\hat{\nu} = \alpha(< 1)$ if p_1 is found in the documents and p_2 is not found there, and is estimated as $\hat{\nu} = 1$ in other cases. In the reevaluation of a valid entry, ν is estimated as $\hat{\nu} = \beta$ if none of the patterns is not found in the documents, and is estimated $\hat{\nu} = 0$ in other case. The values of α and β are also estimated by using the learning data described in Section 4.2.

In this reevaluation, we need the retrieved documents that contain both the target variant and its canonical form. We can use MEDLINE documents, but there is little paraphrase information there because the texts in the MEDLINE database are abstracts of the fruit of research and the length of each text entry is usually limited to a fixed size. Therefore we use the documents retrieved using a Web search engine for the reevaluation.

4   Outline of the System and the Experiment

In this section, we present the processing step of the invalid dictionary detection system and describe the data and parameters used in the evaluation experiments.

4.1   Invalid Dictionary Entry Detection System

Based on the methods described in the previous section, we set up a system to detect invalid entries in the dictionary. Figure 1 shows an overview of the system. In this system, we first evaluate the dictionary entry based on the frequency information (FC) as described in Section 3.2. In this evaluation, we used the MEDLINE documents published from January 1996 to December 2004 for the test corpus. The size of test corpus is 3,755,182 documents. By using the paraphrase information described in Section 3.3, we reevaluate the entries that were previously evaluated as invalid (WP1) or as valid (WP2). For the paraphrase pattern search, we needed documents containing both the variant and its canonical form. For these documents, we use the first 20 documents retrieved by using the Google APIs[1].

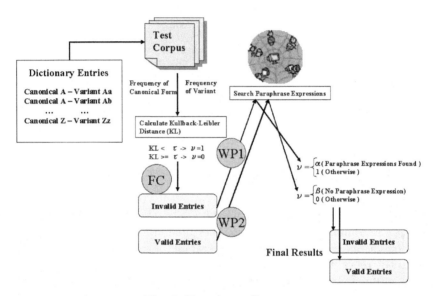

Fig. 1. Experiment System

4.2   Data and Parameter Setting

For the experiment, we constructed the dictionary using the information in Entrez Gene, UMLS, and Swiss-Prot. From the dictionary, we used the dictionary entries for 200 canonical forms that were Official Symbols of Entrez Gene. On average, each canonical form had almost six variants, resulting in 1,137 dictionary entries consisting of a variant and its canonical form.

For these dictionary entries, four domain experts assigned one of 3 evaluation scores (0: valid, 0.5: invalid in some cases, 1: invalid). Table 2 shows examples of the evaluation. For each entry, we calculate ν as $\nu = \frac{1}{n} \sum_{i=1}^{n} s_j$ where n is the number of experts and s_j is the j-th expert's score for the invalidity. Table 2 also shows the values of ν and the resulting risk score for the entries.

We divided these dictionary entries with risk scores into two groups: learning data and evaluation data. We used 50 canonical forms and their variants for the

---

[1] http://www.google.com/apis/

Table 2. Example of the Evaluation by Domain Experts and the Risk Score

canonical form	variant	expert 1	expert 2	expert 3	expert 4	ν	f_S	$rs(S)$
Spna2	brain	1	1	1	1	1.000	645985	0.984
Dhfr2	Dihydrofolate reductase	0.5	0	0.5	0.5	0.375	4170	0.476
STMN1	leukemia-associated gene	1	1	0	0.5	0.625	13	0.346

learning data (288 entries). We used the 150 canonical forms and their variants for the evaluation data (849 entries). Using the learning data, we estimated the parameters used in the invalidity detection methods such that $\tau = 2.0 \times 10^{-4}$, $\alpha = 0.40$, and $\beta = 0.43$. Using these estimated parameters, we set up the invalid dictionary entry detection system and investigated how many invalid entries in the evaluation data were correctly cleaned up.

5   Results

In the experiments, we estimated the risk score for each entry in the evaluation data, detected the invalid entries, and compared them with those based on the experts' evaluation. Table 3 shows the precision, recall, and F-value for each method. In Table 3, FC shows the results using only the KL-distance, FC+WP1 includes the reevaluations of the invalid entry using the FC results, FC+WP2 includes the reevaluations of the valid entries using the FC results, and FC+WP1+WP2 includes the reevaluations of the both the invalid and valid entries using the FC results. By considering the reevaluations of the invalid entries in the results of FC, the precision is improved but the recall and the F-value are not improved. On the other hand, by considering the reevaluations of the valid entries in the results of FC, both the recall and the F-value are improved.

Table 4 shows the invalid dictionary entries detected by the evaluation based on the KL-distance between the occurrence frequency distributions of the canonical word and its variant. For each canonical form and variant, the value in the parenthesis shows the frequency in the test collection that we used for the calculations of the KL-distances. From this table, it can be seen that variants that are not common nouns but that frequently appears in the test corpus are detected as invalid entries. Though whether or not the variant frequently appears depends on the frequency of the canonical form and we cannot use the threshold for the invalidity evaluation, we can detect the invalid entries by using the distance between the appearance distributions.

Table 3. Precision and Recall in each Method

	Precision	Recall	F-value
FC	0.680	0.741	0.709
FC+WP1	0.692	0.716	0.704
FC+WP2	0.660	0.781	0.715
FC+WP1+WP2	0.667	0.776	0.717

Table 4. Examples of the Invalid Entries

canonical form (frequency)	variant (frequency)	canonical form (frequency)	variant (frequency)
INS (420)	insulin (37,335)	da (582)	dark (9,708)
rb (66)	rabbit (20,790)	Axin (158)	Ki (3,674)
IRF6 (18)	LPS (14,011)	CALCA (13)	KC (751)
INSR (12)	IR (9,217)	PBL2 (5)	p130 (563)
LEP (178)	obese (12,089)	IRF6 (18)	PPS (739)
ec (55)	ectopic (7,906)	DDR1 (33)	NEP (606)

Table 5. Examples of the Reevaluation Entries

canonical form (frequency)	variant (frequency)	$rs(S)$ (reevaluated)	$rs(S)$ (expert)
NOS1 (95)	nNOS (1,631)	0.000	0.263
AICDA (4)	AID (260)	0.384	0.316

Table 6. Examples of the Reevaluation Entries

canonical form (frequency)	variant (frequency)	$rs(S)$ (reevaluated)	$rs(S)$ (expert)
Li (2,545))	lines (2,032)	0.466	0.616
APP (2,096)	AAA (2,175))	0.468	0.714
FGFR (405)	H5 (455)	0.418	0.637

Table 5 and Table 6 show the result of the reevaluations of the evaluation based on the KL-distances between the occurrence distributions. In these tables, there are the final risk scores estimated by the system and the risk scores based on the experts' evaluations. Table 5 shows the entries reevaluated as valid because we can find paraphrase expressions in the documents containing the canonical form and the variant. For NOS1, we can find paraphrase patterns p_1 and p_2 and therefore we estimate $\hat{\nu} = 0$ and regard it as valid entry though it was regarded as invalid by the KL-distance-based evaluation. Table 6 shows the entries reevaluated as invalid because we cannot find any paraphrase expression for the valid entry based on the KL-distances. This shows that we can detect the invalid dictionary entries whose canonical forms and variants have almost same frequencies by considering the paraphrase expression extractions. For example, though AAA is registered as one of the Gene aliases for APP in Entrez Gene, AAA is also the name of protein superfamily that is not related to APP. Therefore, we should regard AAA to be an invalid variant of APP because we get many unrelated documents on APP by identifying AAA with APP.

6   Discussion

From the results shown, though it was found that the invalid dictionary entry detection is improved by considering the paraphrase expression finding for the canonical forms and their variants, the differences in the results are small. One of the reasons is that the valid entries are overlooked by the paraphrase expression finding in the results evaluated as invalid in FC. For example, SNAP-25 appears more frequently in the test corpus than its canonical form SNAP25 and is regarded as invalid when using FC. SNAP-25 is one of the spelling variation of the canonical form and should be reevaluated as valid, but usually there are no paraphrase expressions for such spelling variations. Therefore such dictionary entries are finally reevaluated as invalid in the proposed methods. In this case, we lose a lot of useful information about SNAP25. For this problem, we need to expand the canonical form, generate suitable spelling variations, and confirm whether or not the variant is in the spelling variations. A method was proposed to learn the probabilistic rules for generating variants from the raw texts [10]. It was reported that the term aggregation using only the dictionary search was not sufficient [4], because not all of the spelling variations in the dictionary can be generated from the external resources, but by applying the spelling variation generation method to the dictionary entries modified by the proposed methods, we can get a dictionary that has much richer entries. In the paraphrase expression finding, we use only simple string matching to the prepared patterns. There are other variation for the expressions such as "... leptin *gene* (LEP) ". Therefore we think that we need a method to generate the paraphrase expression patterns using the learning data. Improvement of the detection methods using the paraphrase expression will be some of our future work.

In the FC approach, we evaluated an entry as invalid when the KL-distance was larger than the threshold. Therefore, we also evaluated the entry as invalid when the frequency of the variant was much smaller than that of its canonical form and then set $\hat{\nu} = 1.0$. In such a case, the estimated risk score is not large because of the small frequency. However we need to avoid evaluating such an entry as invalid in the FC. We think that by using some heuristics about the frequency of the variant, we can avoid this problem and improve the results of the FC.

7   Conclusion

In this paper, we described an automatically generated dictionary from external resources frequently used for the biomedical text mining and pointed out that there are some invalid entries that have negative impacts on the text mining function such as the calculations of distributions of the keyword frequencies, and we need to exclude such invalid words from the dictionary. To solve this problem, we defined the invalid dictionary entries that should be excluded for the keyword frequency calculation in the text mining and proposed the methods to detect such invalid entries. To detect the invalid dictionary entries, we proposed a method based on the KL-distances between the frequency distributions of a variant and its canonical form, and a method using paraphrase expression extraction in the documents that contain the variant and its canonical form.

As a result, it was found that we can improve both recall and F-value by considering these two detection methods. In the real text mining application, we usually check the list of entries with their risk scores and decide on the invalid dictionary entries from that list. Therefore it is expected that we can easily detect almost all of the invalid entries that have negative impacts on the calculations of the keyword frequencies. For further improvement we need to introduce some heuristics for the evaluations based on the KL-distance. We also need to introduce a suitable spelling variation generation system and modify the paraphrase expression finding. These are our future projects.

Acknowledgement

We would like to thank Daisuke Minegishi and Hiroshi Kitajima for their evaluations of the dictionary entries. We are grateful to Hiroyuki Koiwa and Kohichi Takeda for their continuing support. We also appreciate the valuable comments from reviewers.

References

1. B. Boeckmann, A. Bairoch, R. Apweiler, M.C. Blatter, A. Estreicher, E. Gasteiger, et al. SWISS-PROT protein knowledgebase and its supplement TrEMBL in 2003. *Nucleic Acids Research*, 31(1), 365–370, 2003.
2. B.L. Humphrey and H.M. Schoolman. The Unified Medical Language System: An Informatics Research Collaboration. *Journal of the American Medical Informatics Association*, 5(1), 1–11, 1998.
3. A. Koike and T. Takagi. Gene/ Protein/ Family Name Recognition in Biomedical Literature. *HLT-NAACL 2004 Workshop: BioLink 2004, Linking Biological Literature, Ontologies and Databases*, 9–16, 2004.
4. M. Krauthammer and G. Nenadic. Term Identification in the Biomedical Literature. *Journal of Biomedical Informatics*, 37(6), 512–526, 2004.
5. H. Liu, Z. Hu, J. Zhang and C. Wu. BioThesaurus: A Web-Based Thesaurus of Protein and Gene Names. *Bioinformatics*, 22(1) 103–105, 2006.
6. T. Nasukawa and T. Nagano. Text analysis and knowledge mining system. *IBM System Journal*, 40(4), 967-984, 2001.
7. K.D. Pruitt and D.R. Maglott. RefSeq and LocusLink: NCBI gene-centered resources. *Nucleic Acids Research*, 29(1), 137–140, 2001.
8. A.S. Schwartz and M.A. Hearst A Simple Algorithm for Identifying Abbreviation Definitions in Biomedical Text *Proceeding of the Pac. Symp. Biocomput.*, 451–462, 2003.
9. H. Shatkay and R. Feldman. Mining the Biomedical Literature in the Genomic Era: An Overview. *Journal of Computational Biology*, 10(6), 821–855, 2003.
10. Y. Tsuruoka and J. Tsujii. Probabilistic Term Variant Generator for Biomedical Terms. *Proceeding of the SIGIR 2003*, 167–173, 2003.
11. O. Tuason, L. Chen, H. Liu, J.A.Blake and C. Friedman. Biological nomenclatures: a source of lexical knowledge and ambiguity. *Proceeding of the Pac. Symp. Biocomput.*, 238–249, 2004.
12. N. Uramoto, H. Matsuzawa, T. Nagano, A. Murakami, H. Takeuchi and K. Takeda. A Text-Mining System for Knowledge Discovery from Biomedical Documents. *IBM System Journal*, 43(3), 516-533, 2004.

Automated Identification of Protein Classification and Detection of Annotation Errors in Protein Databases Using Statistical Approaches

Kang Ning[1] and Hon Nian Chua[2]

[1] School of Computing, National University of Singapore,
3 Science Drive 2, Singapore, 117543
ningkang@comp.nus.edu.sg
[2] National University of Singapore
g0306417@nus.edu.sg

Abstract. Because of the importance of proteins in life sciences, biologists have put great effort to elucidate their structures, functions and expression profiles to help us understand their roles in living cells in the past few decades. Currently, protein databases are widely used by biologists. Hence it is critical that the information that researcher work with should be as accurate as possible. However, the sizes of these databases are increasing rapidly, and existing protein databases are already known to contain annotation errors. In this paper, we investigate the reason why protein databases possess mis-annotated sequence data. Then, by using some statistical approaches, we derive a method to automatically filter and assess the reliability of the data from databases. This is important to provide accurate information to researchers and will help reduce further errors in annotation resulting from existed mis-annotated sequence data. Our initial experiments proved our theoretical findings, and show that our methods can effectively detect the mis-annotated sequence data.

1 Introduction

With the improvement of sequencing technology in life sciences, protein sequence data is accumulated in an astonishing rate within the past several years. Thus developing a computational method for automatic protein annotation becomes very crucial in order to keep up with the fast pace of sequence data generation [1].

Automatic large-scale protein classification and annotation attempt to infer functional characterization of unknown proteins or its domains based on the sequence similarity with some well-annotated protein in protein database [2]. Some web-based program was developed for automatic annotation of any kind of protein sequence with biological information, like PANDORA (Protein ANnotation Diagram ORiented Analysis) [3]. However, the potential risk of this method is when it tries to derive annotation information from proteins with multiple domains, wrong domain information may be annotated for querying sequence. Another source of annotation error may be produced from the best-matching

E.G. Bremer et al. (Eds.): KDLL 2006, LNBI 3886, pp. 123–138, 2006.

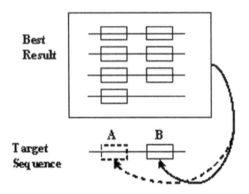

Fig. 1. A misclassification example

domain is not fully characterized or well-annotated. Once an error existed in a database, it tends to propagate because it may be cited or referred by other annotations. The error will spread from that point to various entry in a database or entered into other database.

Figure 1 shows an example of misclassification of protein class. The query sequence contain only a domain B. The hits returned from BLAST [4] represent a cluster of proteins that contain more domain A than domain B. Thus target protein may be mis-annotated with domain A rather than domain B.

An example of protein with such mis-classification is $inosine - 5'monophos - phatedehydrogenase(IMPDH)$ [5]. There were several $non - IMPDH$ protein sequences misclassified as $IMPDH$ protein in the major protein database such as $SWISS - PROT$ and $GenBank$ and was only recently rectified. It was largely due to the presence of the CBS domain which was not unique to $IMPDH$ protein but present in many $IMPDH$ protein. Many misclassified protein also propagated into secondary databases [1].

Recently, there is an increasing concern about the estimation of misclassification errors[6,19]. In this paper, we intended to derive a set of methods to automatically filter and assess the reliability of the data from databases, by using some statistical approaches.

There are statistical approaches have been tried by some other researchers [19]. In [19], the researchers used C4.5 data mining algorithm for the annotation of keywords on SWISS-PROT protein sequences. In this paper, we have also used the statistical approaches, but we have used the Naive Bayesian algorithms for the proteins sequences classifications and error detections.

Our preliminary approach include multiple sequence alignment on search results to identify similar regions that does not apply to all sequences being compared and from these suspicious region do further search to confirm these suspicions. As protein sequences are relatively much shorter than nucleotide sequences (a few tens to a few thousand amino acids), multiple sequence alignment may be feasible to conduct an analysis within reasonable time. An illustration of this approach is in Figure 2.

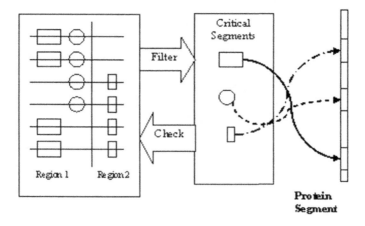

Fig. 2. The local alignment approach

Another approach is to identify a key protein sequence or domain(s) that uniquely identifies a family of protein. These highly conserved regions perform critical functions and even a single mutation on that region may cause the demise of the host organism. These domain sequences can be derived from annotations of protein sequence in the database or through pairwise multiple alignments of protein sequences that are most likely to be of the same family. Such sequences may be retrieved using BLASTp [4] and analyzing several of the top hits' sequence. Upon deriving this key protein sequence(s), we can then do local alignments on a sequence to determine if it belongs to this family. We have implemented an tool (interface) to validate our theoretical findings. This tool will be an interface through which a user can search for similar protein sequences by providing a sequence as input.

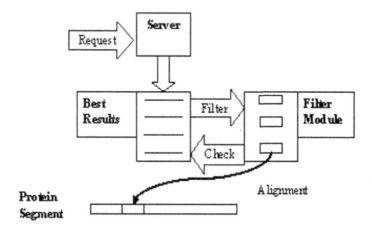

Fig. 3. The outline of the place and function of the filtering tool

Refer to Figure 3 for an outline of how this tool (interface) is going to be incorporated into existing databases. When searching for sequences similar to a target protein sequence, the target protein is sent to the interface, which will send the request to the database server (e.g. BLAST). Upon receiving the results, the interface does a post query analysis on the results to identify possible misclassification or mis-annotation and to provide the user with more information of similar regions and how likely the target sequence is to be from a certain family.

2   Related Works

Currently, various projects were initiated for automatic protein annotation. Some researchers have begun to notice the potential errors that may occur from traditional computational annotation approach and improve their program by introducing some modules to filter out false annotations. [1][5].

Since large-scale protein annotation relies much on the classification on the known proteins, it is important to understand the standard and rationale of protein classification. We will describe some of them briefly.

Hierarchical families of proteins – superfamilies/families. The Protein Information Resource (PIR)[7] serves as an integrated public resource of functional annotation of protein data to support genomic/proteomic research and scientific discovery. The PIR produces the PIR-International Protein Sequence Database (PSD), the major annotated protein sequence database in the public domain containing about 250,000 proteins. The superfamily/family classification is a unique characteristic of the PIR-PSD [8]. It provides complete and non-overlapping clustering of proteins based on global sequence similarity.

Families of protein domains. Pfam [9] is a large collection of protein multiple sequence alignments and profile hidden Markov models. Pfam contains 3071 families, which match 69% of proteins in SWISS-PROT and TrEMBL [10]. Pfam also utilize structural data to ensure Pfam families correspond with structural domains, and to improve domain-based annotation.

Sequence motifs or conserved regions. PROSITE [11] is a database of protein families and domains, using a method of identifying what is the function of uncharacterized proteins translated from genomic or cDNA sequences. It consists of biologically significant sites, patterns and profiles that help to reliably identify to which known protein family (if any) a new sequence belongs.

　　PRINTS [12] is more or less similar to PROSITE, but it is only a compendium of protein fingerprints.

Structural classes. Examples are SCOP [13] and CATH [14].

Integrations of various family classifications. One example is iProClass [15].

Discussions about these works
Although there are so many kinds of databases using various kinds of classification criteria and annotation approaches, they are mostly consistent. In most

cases, sequence similarity can lead to structural similarity and functional similarity, so given a normal protein, you can usually get the right annotation no matter which database or which strategy you are using. Meanwhile, each of them improves the identification of proteins that are difficult to characterize based on pairwise alignments, and also reflects the underlying gene families.

While each of these databases is useful for particular needs, no classification scheme is by itself adequate for addressing all genomic annotation needs, especially for discovering the error annotation. Besides, many database users rely on searching a comprehensive database for the best-scoring retrieved matches in making identifications of unknown proteins. There are several problems with this approach.

Generally, the common sequence searching algorithms (BLAST[16], FASTA[17]) find best-scoring similarities; however, the similarity may involve only parts of the query and target molecules. Besides, the retrieved similarity may be to a known domain that is tangential to the main function of the protein or to a region with compositional similarity.

More over, annotation in the searched databases is at best inconsistent and incomplete and at worst misleading or erroneous, having been based on partial or weak similarity. Users need to realize that entries in a comprehensive database may be under-identified, over-identified or mis-identified.

In many cases a more thorough and time-consuming analysis is needed to reveal the most probable functional assignments. Factors that may be relevant, in addition to presence or absence of domains, motifs, or functional residues, include similarity or potential similarity of three-dimensional structures, proximity of genes, metabolic capacities of the organisms, and evolutionary history of the protein as deduced from aligned sequences.

Faced with these problems, we turn to statistics. Statistical methods are especially suitable in cases where lots of hidden variables exist for the complex relationships among many different datasets in the system. In the following part, we will show how to solve some of the problems, for example, to recognize the old, incomplete and even erroneous annotations, during our annotation of the new protein.

3   Statistical Approaches

In order to address the problems we have discussed, we need to find techniques that can detect inconsistency in annotations swiftly without involving tedious and time-consuming investigation and analysis by the user. Realizing that deterministic approaches are not likely to work well due to the complexity of protein classification and the need for a reasonably fast solution, we adopt a heuristic method on the statistical basis to quickly identify regions related to protein function and determine their existence in various related sequences.

The statistical basis is the naive Bayesian Classifier. The naive Bayesian classifier is a simple approach to represent, use and learn probabilistic knowledge. It is a method with clear semantics, and it can be used in supervised induction tasks, in which the performance goal is to accurately predict the class of test instances and in which the training instances include class information. The naive Bayesian classifier is a simplified form of Bayesian network. The term *naive* relies on 2 simplification assumptions. It assumes that the predictive attribute are conditionally independent of the classes, and there is no hidden or latent attributes that influence the prediction process.

The naive assumptions make very efficient algorithm for both classification and learning. Let G be the random variable representing the class of an instance, and let S be a vector variable denoting the observed attributes values. Also, let g represents a particular class label, and s represents a particular observed attributes value vector. The probability of a sequence to have a certain annotation, P(G=g—S=s) by Bayes' rule is:

$$P(G = g|S = s) = \frac{P(G = g)P(S = s|G = g)}{P(S = s)}$$

Thus, the most probable class can be predicted. The vector value $X = x$ represents the event that $X_1 = x_1 \wedge X_2 = x_2 \wedge \ldots X_k = x_k$. Since the event is a conjunction of attribute values, and because these attributes are assumed to be conditionally independent, we have

$$P(S = s|G = g) = P(\bigwedge_i S_i = s_i|G = g)$$

$$= \prod_i P(S_i = s_i|G = g)$$

The classifier assigns annotations to sequences by taking the maximum $P(S = s|G = g)$ value, on calculating all of the probable annotations. $P(S = s)$, the probability of finding annotations, is constant(independent of class) and can be excluded. Thus, the naive Bayesian classification is equivalent to Maximum A Posteriori estimate(MAP)[19]. When the a priori probabilities of finding the different classes are equal, i.e., $P(G = g)$ for different g's are qual, the procedure is equivalent to the Maximum Likelihood estimate(ML).

The naive Bayesian classifier can be used to accurately annotate the protein sequences. It can achieve this performance goal by two directions. First, by annotating the sequence using highly conserved regions, those mis-annotated protein sequences may have low support to be annotated to the wrong annotation. Second, by annotating the sequence using suspect sequences (sequences which are less likely to be in the protein sequence with the specific annotation),the mis-annotated protein sequences have high probability to be detected.

In this project, we have developed a statistical approach by combining local alignment and statistical method to identify conserved regions that are likely to determine functions and hence classification of proteins. From an input sequence, we are able to estimate such conserved regions in similar sequences as well as the presence or absence of these regions in these sequences. Using this result, we can

– Infer the classification of the input sequence based on the presence or absence of different regions in comparison to similar sequences
– Detect possible annotation errors in the database if the results of similarly annotated sequences are inconsistent
– Identify highly conserved regions that provide functionality in protein

It is interesting to note that as the online sequence analysis tools become more and more powerful, the statistical tests can be done fairly well by the use of those tools, together with a little analysis done on the local machine.

The technique that we developed comprises 3 main parts

– Find protein sequences similar to input sequence using local alignment and find the longest of these sequences. Let this longest sequence be x. Find protein sequences similar to x, again using local alignment
– Among these sequences, group highly similar sequences together and apply statistical methods to estimate highly conserved regions. Compare these regions among different groups and for overlapping regions, find the common regions
– Examine all sequences to determine if they contain these regions base on their similarity to the x within the each region

Step 1: Finding Longest Sequence
Transitional errors in protein databases were due to the existence of more than one domains in proteins. When two proteins X and Y are similar to a third protein Z at two separate regions, this give rise to a possibility of associating the two proteins X and Y even though they do not have any correlation.

Hence given an input sequence, we want to find some sequence that is highly likely to contain domains in the input sequence as well as domains that may belong to other sequences since such a case can give rise to transitional annotation errors. The longest sequence above a certain similarity is likely to be such a sequence. Since different proteins can have similar domains, local alignment is the most intuitive way to identify protein with similar domains.

Drawing from these observations, we try to find a sequence that may cause possible errors in annotations by first using BLAST to find protein sequences similar to the input sequence and subsequently retrieving the longest sequence from those sequences that with E-Score above a certain threshold. This threshold is to ensure that the sequence we pick is likely to have at least one similar domain to the input sequence.

Step 2: Estimating Highly Conserved Regions
Domains are subunits of protein that perform specific functions. As these domains are critical to the function of the protein, they are significantly conserved in the evolution process. Hence they are present as highly similar regions in sequences that have similar function.

Base on this concept, we try to estimate possible functional domains by identifying regions that are highly conserved in different protein sequences. Using the Suspect sequence from step 1, we perform a BLAST query to get sequences that are similar to the Suspect sequence base on local alignment. By identifying regions that are similar to different sequences, we try to identify possible domains.

Using the E-score from BLAST as a metric, we group these sequences into similar groups according to their similarity at regions that match the Suspect sequence. Within each group, we count the number of sequences that match each amino acid in the Suspect sequence at its position in the Suspect sequence. If this count is large relative to the number of sequence in the group, then that particular amino acid is likely to be part of a domain.

To improve the sensitivity, we included the following steps

- From available protein domain databases we know that determining existence of protein domains in sequences are based on similarity and not exact match. Hence, we allow for mismatches up to a certain number of amino acids
- We exclude such short regions to remove false positives
- We link short matching regions to form regions of at least 20 amino acids
- Exclude sequences exceedingly similar to the Suspect sequence as such sequences may be the same protein as the Suspect sequence

Combining the regions derived from every group and finding common regions whenever there are overlapping regions, we get our final set of highly conserved regions (HCRs).

Step 3: Determining the existence of HCRs
After estimating highly conserved regions, we have to determine if a given protein sequence contains each of these regions. Using the principle of hamming distance, we assign a simple similarity score by counting the number of amino acid in that sequence that matches the Suspect sequence in its position within that region, and dividing this by the length of that region.

$$S = \frac{m}{n}$$

where S is the similarity score, m is the number of amino acid matches with the Suspect sequence within the region and n is the length of the region.

S is a value from 0 to 1 and is proportional to the similarity of a sequence to the Suspect sequence within the region. Using a threshold $0 < t < 1$, we report that the sequence contains that domain if $S > t$.

4   Results and Discussions

Using the above approach, we are able to get rather promising results. We have tried Bayesian method on protein classification, and results are satisfactory.

For the classification of protein sequences based on naive Bayesian method, we have chosen the protein sequences from Rodentia, Rattus, Alphavirus, Hepevirus and Drosophila organisms from SWISS-PROT[10] database. To simulate the real

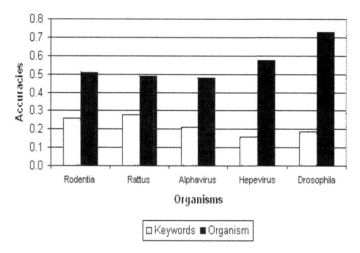

Fig. 4. The classification accuracies of protein sequences by naive Bayesian method

protein seuqences classification, we have set the length of protein sequences to be 100, and the length of domains is set to be 9. These are appropriate values based on previous findings. We have used the 10-fold cross-validation test on the sequences data to evaluate the accuracies.

Part of the classification results are illustrated in Figure 4. The organism, as well as more detailed keywords accuracies are illustrated.

We can observe that although the accuracies for keywords classification are not so high, the accuracies for classification of organisms are quite resealable. Since the accuracies of naive Bayesian classification is accurate, we can confidently use this method for the classification of more complicated protein sequences and detection of annotation errors.

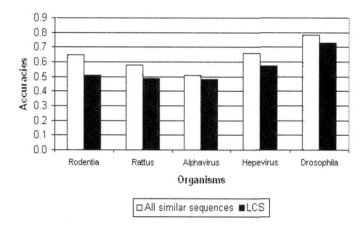

Fig. 5. The comparisons of classification accuracies of protein sequences based on all similar sequences against LCS

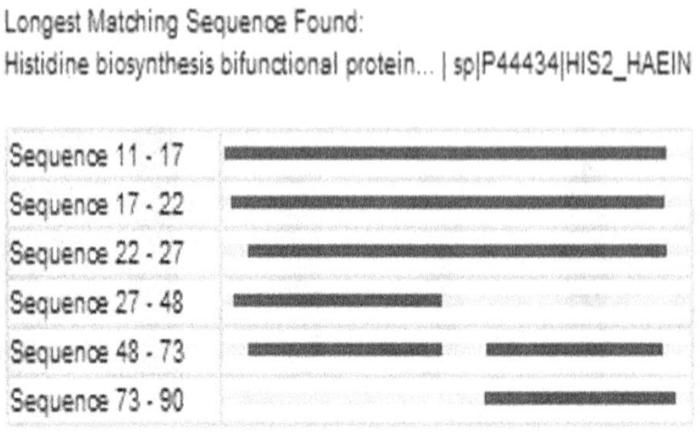

Longest Matching Sequence Found:

Histidine biosynthesis bifunctional protein... | sp|P44434|HIS2_HAEIN

Sequence 11 - 17	████████████████████
Sequence 17 - 22	████████████████████
Sequence 22 - 27	███████████████████
Sequence 27 - 48	████████████
Sequence 48 - 73	████████ ████████
Sequence 73 - 90	███████████

Fig. 6. Highly Conserved Region for different group of sequences. HCRs are in dark color.

More over, we have done experiments to show that the step 1 of our approach (only take Longest Common Subsequence (LCS)) has comparable performance to the simple method that take in all of the similar sequences of the input sequence. The comparison results are shown in 5.

The little differences between them clearly shows that the step 1 has reasonable performance. This is probably due to the fact that we have taken the Longest Common Subsequence (LCS) in step 1, and most of the common domains are in this region.

Here we present two case studies in details to illustrate the results and application of our techniques. In our implementation, we use BLASTp [4] on the SWISS-PROT[10] database.

Automated identification

In this case, we show that our technique correctly identify conserved regions as well as their existence in sequences similar to a input sequence and consequently provides a basis to infer the family of the input sequence.

Using $O30723$ *Phosphoribosyl − ATP* pyrophosphatase as the input, we get $p|P44434|HIS2_H AEIN$, Histidine biosynthesis bifunctional protein as the longest matching sequence found. After doing a BLAST on this sequence and grouping similar sequences from the results, we derive highly conserved regions for each group. We allow up to 10 mismatches in regions and set 20 as the minimum size for a region. Figure 6 illustrates the regions found for the different groups of sequences.

Breaking overlapped regions into separate regions, we get three regions that are likely to be domains. See Figure 7.

Domain 0 (13 - 102)	██████████████
Domain 1 (103 - 123)	███
Domain 2 (124 - 207)	████████████

Fig. 7. Resulting Estimated Likely Domains. Likely domains are in dark color.

Model	Seq-from	Seq-to	HMM-from	HMM-to	Score	E-value	Alignment	Description
!! PRA-CH	18	92	1	77	175.7	8.2e-50	glocal	Phosphoribosyl-AMP cyclohydrolase

Fig. 8. pFam search results using regions found by our approach(a)

We examine the regions found by doing a search using Pfam. By performing a search in Pfam on these regions, we discovered that Region 1 (13-102) coincides with $Phosphoribosyl - AMP$ cyclohydrolase and Region 3 (124-207) coincides with $Phosphoribosyl - ATP$ pyrophosphatase. Refer to Figure 8 and Figure 9.

The last step of our technique analyzes all sequences similar to the longest sequence and reports the existence of the regions found earlier in each sequence. Refer to Figure 10 for a tabulated result from this step. All $Phosphoribosyl - ATP$ pyrophosphatase sequences are reported to contain Region 1, which was verified earlier to be the ATP pyrophosphatase domain. Similarly, all $Phosphoribosyl - AMP$ cyclohydrolase sequences are reported to contain Region 3, which was verified earlier to be the AMP cyclohydrolase domain.

There were also Histidine biosynthesis sequences in the results. These sequences contain both Region 1 and Region 3. Upon looking at the annotation of P00815 Histidine biosynthesis trifunction protein, we can see that it contains both $Phosphoribosyl - ATP$ pyrophosphatase and $Phosphoribosyl - AMP$ cyclohydrolase. Refer to Figure 11.

By increasing the minimum size for regions, Region 2, which does not contain any protein domain, is removed. See Figure 12.

Hence we can see that our method correctly identify two functional domains and also correctly determine their existence in sequences similar to the input sequence. Since the $Phosphoribosyl - ATP$ pyrophosphatase region is found in the input sequence, we can infer that the input sequence is a $Phosphoribosyl - ATP$ pyrophosphatase protein. We know that this is true since we used a $Phosphoribosyl - ATP$ pyrophosphatase protein as the input sequence. Hence the inference using the results is accurate.

Detection of errors
We know that $sp|Q58069|Y653_{M}ETJA$ $Hypothetical$ $protein$ $MJ0653$ is annotated in previous versions of GenPept to contain inosine-5'-monophosphate dehydrogenase (IMPDH). See Figure 13.

We use $sp|Q58069|Y653_{M}ETJA$ Hypothetical protein MJ0653 with our technique introduced earlier. We get a number of highly conserved regions as illustrated in Figure 14.

Model	Seq-from	Seq-to	HMM-from	HMM-to	Score	E-value	Alignment	Description
!! PRA-PH	1	84	1	95	146.0	7e-41	glocal	Phosphoribosyl-ATP pyrophosphohydrolase

Fig. 9. pFam search results using regions found by our approach(b)

Protein		13 - 102	103 - 123	124 - 207
sp|O30723|HIS2_RHOCA Phosphoribosyl-ATP pyrophosphatase (PRA-PH)	Pfam	No	No	Yes
sp|P26722|HIS2_AZOBR Phosphoribosyl-ATP pyrophosphatase (PRA-PH)	Pfam	No	No	Yes
sp|P50935|HIS2_RHOSH Phosphoribosyl-ATP pyrophosphatase (PRA-PH)	Pfam	No	No	Yes
sp|Q8YE38|HIS2_BRUME Phosphoribosyl-ATP pyrophosphatase (PRA-PH)	Pfam	No	No	Yes
sp|Q8UJ91|HIS2_AGRT5 Phosphoribosyl-ATP pyrophosphatase (PRA-PH)	Pfam	No	No	Yes
sp|P58834|HIS2_METAC Phosphoribosyl-ATP pyrophosphatase (PRA-PH)	Pfam	No	No	Yes
sp|Q8PUG2|HIS2_METMA Phosphoribosyl-ATP pyrophosphatase (PRA-PH)	Pfam	No	'o	v
sp|O9°° ···· ··· ···vl-ATP ···· ···RA-··.		···		
····HIS2 ···· . ·iosphori··· ····rophosphatase (PRA-PH)	Pfam		I,	Yes
····Q9EWK0|HIS2_STRCO Phosphoribosyl-ATP pyrophosphatase (PRA-PH)	Pfam	No	No	Yes
sp|P58835|HIS2_METKA Phosphoribosyl-ATP pyrophosphatase (PRA-PH)	Pfam	No	No	Yes
sp|Q97KH7|HIS3_CLOAB Phosphoribosyl-AMP cyclohydrolase (PRA-CH)	Pfam	Yes	No	No
sp|O28329|HIS3_ARCFU Phosphoribosyl-AMP cyclohydrolase (PRA-CH)	Pfam	Yes	No	No
sp|Q9S2U1|HIS3_STRCO Phosphoribosyl-AMP cyclohydrolase (PRA-CH)	Pfam	Yes	No	No
sp|Q8TS96|HIS3_METAC Phosphoribosyl-AMP cyclohydrolase (PRA-CH)	Pfam	Yes	No	No
sp|Q8XV86|HIS3_RALSO Phosphoribosyl-AMP cyclohydrolase (PRA-CH)	Pfam	Yes	No	No
sp|Q8PVF°···· ···TMA Ph·· ···svl-AMP cyc·° ··· ··(P··	°fam			No
····sc|HIS3_METK··. ···sphoribosyl-A··. ···yclohydrolase (, ··.CH)	P··,	Yes	No	.
sp|Q50837|HIS3_METVA Phosphoribosyl-AMP cyclohydrolase (PRA-CH)	Pfam	Yes	No	No
sp|P07685|HIS2_NEUCR Histidine biosynthesis trifunctional protei...	Pfam	Yes	Yes	Yes
sp|Q12670|HIS2_SACBA Histidine biosynthesis trifunctional protei...	Pfam	Yes	Yes	Yes
sp|P00815|HIS2_YEAST Histidine biosynthesis trifunctional protei...	Pfam	Yes	Yes	Yes
sp|O13471|HIS2_KLULA Histidine biosynthesis trifunctional protei...	Pfam	Yes	Yes	Yes
sp|P45353|HIS2_PICPA Histidine biosynthesis trifunctional protei...	Pfam	Yes	Yes	Yes
sp|O74712|HIS2_CANAL Histidine biosynthesis trifunctional protei...	Pfam	Yes	Yes	Yes
sp|P44434|HIS2_HAEIN Histidine biosynth ··is bifunctional protein...	Pfam	Y-	Yes	Yes
sp|Q9CLI°·· °ASMU Histidine b· ··· hifunctional ·· ··n...	Pfam		Yes	Yes
··· Histidi··				

Fig. 10. Tabulated results showing existence of different regions in each sequence

☐ 1: P00815. Histidine biosynt...[gi:123142]

```
LOCUS       P00815                  799 aa             linear    PLN 15-SEP-2003
DEFINITION  Histidine biosynthesis trifunctional protein [Includes:
            Phosphoribosyl-AMP cyclohydrolase ; Phosphoribosyl-ATP
            pyrophosphohydrolase ; Histidinol dehydrogenase (HDH)].
ACCESSION   P00815
```

Fig. 11. NCBI Annotation for 00815 Histidine biosynthesis trifunction

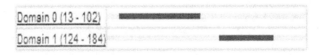

Fig. 12. Resulting Estimated Likely Domains (minimum size of regions increased) are in dark color

Examining these regions using $Pfam$, we found that Region 1, 3, 4, 5 corresponds to the $IMPDH$ domain while Region 2 corresponse to 2 CBS domains (Figure 15).

```
COMMENT     Method: conceptual translation.
FEATURES            Location/Qualifiers
    source          1..194
                    /organism="Methanocaldococcus jannaschii"
                    /db_xref="taxon:2190"
    Protein         1..194
                    /product="inosine-5'-monophosphate dehydrogenase (guaB)"
    CDS             1..194
                    /gene="MJ0653"
                    /coded_by="U67513.1:521..1105"
                    /note="similar to PID:1002715 SP:P50100 percent identity:
                    41.42; identified by sequence similarity; putative"
                    /transl_table=11
```

Fig. 13. Old GenPept entry for Hypothetical Protein MJ0653 (in dark color)

Fig. 14. Regions found with MJ0653 as input sequence

Next we examine the existence of these regions in the various sequences. Figure 16 shows the tabulated results from step 3 of our technique.

We can see that all the $Inosine-5'-monophosphate Dehydrogenase$ proteins has region1, 3, 4 and 5 (IMPDH domain). In fact they also have Region 2 (2 CBS domains) as most $Inosine-5'-monophosphate Dehydrogenase$ proteins also contains 2 CBS domains. MJ0653, however only has the 2 CBS domains (highlighted in black box in Figure 16) and does not contain any IMPDH domain. Hence we can suspect that there is an error in the GenPept annotation.

Model	Seq-from	Seq-to	HMM-from	HMM-to	Score	E-value	Alignment Description
!! CBS	1	47	1	54	12.3	0.12	glocal CBS domain
!! CBS	55	103	1	54	20.3	0.0048	glocal CBS domain

Fig. 15. Region 2 corresponse to 2 CBS domains

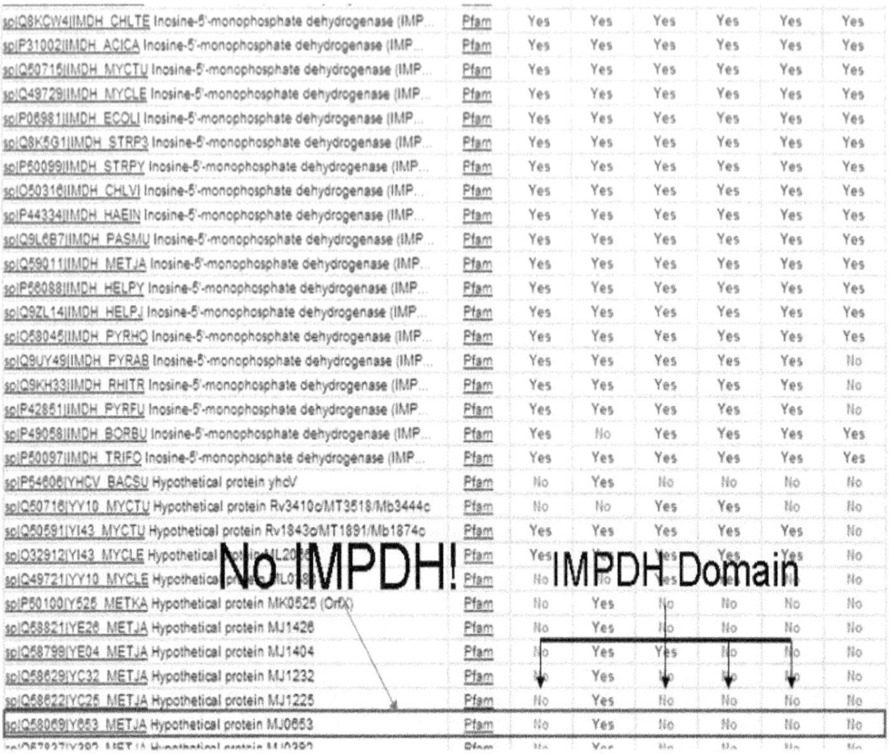

Fig. 16. Tabulated results showing existence of different regions in each sequence

The subsection that this is an annotation error is also mentioned in [6]. The error has been rectified in the current GenPept.

Hence we have shown that this technique is capable of identifying possible errors in annotations. We also showed that this technique can estimate regions likely to be protein domains. We have correctly identified the 2 CBS domains embedded within the IMPDH domain. We can see this by doing a Pfam search using the Suspect sequence. See Figure 17.

Model	Seq-from	Seq-to	HMM-from	HMM-to	Score	E-value	Alignment Description
!! IMPDH	50	527	1	370	643.9	8.9e-191	IMP dehydrogenase / glocal GMP reductase domain
!! CBS	134	190	1	54	36.3	7.5e-08	glocal CBS domain
!! CBS	198	251	1	54	37.5	3.3e-08	glocal CBS domain

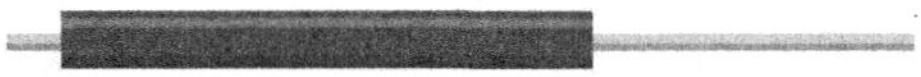

Fig. 17. Embedded CBS domains in an IMPDH domain

This is our first attempt for the detection of errors in protein classification, so we have not measure the accuracy of our error detection method quantitatively, but just tested the method on a few cases.

Though not examined quantitatively, the strength of the method is supported by other research findings. Many of the errors that we have examined have also been verified by other researchers. Actually, based on these cases, we found that our method has good performance, with the error detection accuracy above 80% (details not shown).

5   Conclusion and Future Works

In this paper, we have investigated the reason why protein databases possess mis-annotated sequence data. By using statistical approaches (naive Bayesian), we derived a method to automatically filter and assess the reliability of the data from databases. Our initial experiments proved our theoretical findings, and showed that our methods can effectively detect the mis-annotated sequence data.

There are several places in our method that can be further improved to increase the accuracy of the estimation of conserved regions. They include clustering of similar sequences, and better methods to determine the existence of regions in sequences. We are working on these issues in the future.

Moreover, the naive Bayesian method, being a simple method, maybe not be the best approach for the task. We are currently working on the detection of errors in the annotation of protein sequences using graphical methods, which seems potential from our preliminary studies.

Acknowledgement

We are grateful for anonymous reviewers for their helpful suggestions and advices.

References

1. Wu CH, Huang H, Yeh LS, Barker WC. Protein family classification and functional annotation. *Comput Biol Chem*, 2003 Feb; 27(1):37-47.
2. Abascal F, Valencia A. Automatic annotation of protein function based on family identification. *Proteins*, 2003 Nov 15;53(3):683-92.
3. Kaplan N, Vaaknin A, Linial M. PANDORA: keyword-based analysis of protein sets by integration of annotation sources. *Nucleic Acids Res*, 2003 Oct 1;31(19):5617-26.
4. NCBI BLAST site: *http : //www.ncbi.nlm.nih.gov/BLAST/*
5. Cathy H. Wu and Winona C. Barker. A Family Classification Approach To Functional Annotation Of Proteins. 2003.
6. W. J. Fu, R. J. Carroll, S. Wang. Estimating misclassification error with small samples via bootstrap cross-validation. *Bioinformatics*, doi:10.1093/ bioinformatics/bti294.
7. C. H. Wu, H. Huang, L. Arminski, J. et all. The Protein Information Resource: An integrated public resource of functional annotation of proteins. *Nucleic Acids Research*, 30(1): 35-37, 2002.

8. W. C. Barker, F. Pfeiffer, and D. G. George. Superfamily classification in PIR international protein sequence database. *Methods in Enzymology*, 266:59-71,1996.

9. Bateman, A., Birney, E., Cerruti, L.,Durbin, R., Etwiller, L. et al. (2002). The Pfam protein families database. *Nucl.Acids Res.*, 30,276-80.

10. Bairoch, A., Apweiler, R.(2000). The SWISS-PROT protein sequence database and its supplement TrEMBL in2000. *Nucl. Acids Res.*, 28, 45-48.

11. L. Falquet, M. Pagni, P. Bucher, N. Hulo, C.J.A. Sigritst, K. Hofmann, and A. Bairoch. The PROSITE database, its status in 2002. *Nucleic Acids Research*, 30(1): 235-238, 2002.

12. T. K. Attwood, M. J. Blythe, D. R. Flower, A. Gaulton, J. E. Mabey, N. Maudling, L. McGregor, A. L. Mitchell, G. Moulton, K. Paine, and P. Scordis. PRINTS and PRINTS-S shed light on protein ancestry. *Nucleic Acids Research*, 30: 239-241, 2002.

13. L. Lo Conte, S. E. Brenner, T. J. P. Hubbard, C. Chothia, and A. G. Murzin. SCOP database in 2002: Refinements accommodate structural genomics. *Nucleic Acids Research*, 30: 264-267, 2002.

14. F. M. G. Pearl, N. Martin, J. E. Bray, D. W. A. Buchan, A. P. Harrison, D. Lee, G. A. Reeves, A. J. Shepherd, I. Sillitoe, A. E. Todd, J. M. Thornton, and C. A. Orengo. A rapid classification protocol for the CATH domain database to support structural genomics. *Nucleic Acids Research*, 29: 223-227, 2002.

15. C. H. Wu, C. Xiao, Z. Hou, H. Huang, and W.C. Barker. IProClass: An integrated ,comprehensive, and annotated protein classification database. *Nucleic Acids Research*, 29: 52-54, 2001.

16. S. F. Altschul, W. Gish, W. Miller, E. W. Myers and D. J. Lipman. Basic local alignment tool. *Jounal of Molecular Biology*, 215, 403-410.

17. W. R. Pearson, D. J. Liqman. Improved Tools for Biological Sequence Analysis. *Proc. Natl Acad. Sci. USA*, 85, 2444-2448, 1988.

18. W. J. Fu, R. J. Carroll, S. Wang. Estimating misclassification error with small samples via bootstrap cross-validation. *Bioinformatics*, doi:10.1093/ bioinformatics/bti294.

19. Ernst Kretschmann , Wolfgang Fleischmann and Rolf Apweiler. Automatic rule generation for protein annotation with the C4.5 data mining algorithm applied on SWISS-PROT. *Bioinformatics*, Vol. 17 no. 10 2001.

GetItFull – A Tool for Downloading and Pre-processing Full-Text Journal Articles

Jeyakumar Natarajan[1], Cliff Haines[2], Brian Berglund[2], Catherine DeSesa[3], Catherine J. Hack[1], Werner Dubitzky[1], and Eric G. Bremer[3]

[1] Bioinformatics Research Group, University of Ulster, UK
{j.natarajan, ch.hack, w.dubitzky}@ulster.ac.uk
[2] CTH Technologies, Inc., Oak Brook Terrace, IL USAPSS, Inc, Chicago, IL, USA
{chaines, bberglund}@cthtech.com
[3] Brain Tumor Research Program, Children's Memorial Hospital, and Feinberg School of Medicine, Northwestern University, Chicago, IL, USA
egbremer@northwestern.edu, cdesesa@comcast.net

Abstract. Automated analysis of *full-text* life science research articles and technical documents is becoming increasingly important. In contrast to abstracts, accessing and processing full-text is considerably more complex. GetItFull is a tool for downloading and pre-processing full-text journal articles. GetItFull automatically connects to a journal's Web site, downloads the journal content and performs various commonly used pre-processing steps. The output comprises a structured XML document for each article with tags identifying the various sections and journal information. The output may then be used as the basis for text mining applications or exported to a database for further processing.

1 Introduction

Despite the rapid growth in the volume and number of biological databases available, the scientific literature remains one of the most valuable sources of knowledge to the life scientist. *Knowledge discovery in text* (KDT) comprises a set of technologies which aim *to identify and extract valid, novel and potentially useful information from text* [1]. KDT encompasses three main procedures, namely *information retrieval* (IR), *information extraction* and *text mining* [2]. The aim of IR is to identify relevant documents in response to a query, and thus forms the basis of most KDT processes process [3].

Text mining has been applied successfully to various biological problems including the discovery and characterization of molecular interactions (protein-protein [4,5,6,7,8], gene-protein [9], gene-drug [10]), protein sorting [11,12] and molecular binding [13]. These studies are based on the abstracts of research articles, which represent a readily available resource of highly concentrated information. Whilst fewer studies have used the full-text of articles for their corpus, these studies have shown that full-text documents can provide novel and important information not contained in the article's abstract [14,15,16,17,18]. However, whilst mining of full-text articles can provide more detailed information, the information retrieval step (and subsequent KDT steps) is more

E.G. Bremer et al. (Eds.): KDLL 2006, LNBI 3886, pp. 139–145, 2006.

demanding and complex. This situation is exacerbated by the various formats and organizational structure adopted by different journals.

To overcome these problems and thus make the full-text of biomedical research papers available for text mining, we have designed the downloading and pre-processing tool GetItFull. This tool facilitates a seamless downloading of journals and performs common pre-processing tasks to produce an XML file for each research article. The output may then be used as the basis for text mining applications or exported to a database or other electronic information system for further processing and archiving.

2 System Description

2.1 Overview

The full-texts of research articles are widely available via journal Web sites in HTML and/or PDF format. GetItFull is a Windows-based application tool which uses the Microsoft Web Browser Control [19], an ActiveX control in Microsoft® Visual Studio 6.0 to connect to Internet Explorer DOM interface to navigate and download articles from the journal Web sites using a user-supplied URL address. The system's components and the main processing steps are illustrated in Figure 1.

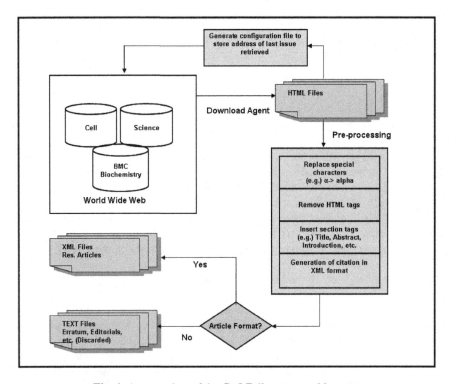

Fig. 1. An overview of the GetItFull system architecture

2.2 Scripting Language

GetItFull provides a scripting mechanism to define downloading and processing tasks. Instructions for writing and modifying scripts are included in the GetItFull software documentation. It is similar to HTML scripting with functions such as <READ>, <WRITE>, <MOVE>, <DO>, and <LOOP> allowing users to read and write to any data source, as well as reformatting text and instigating control structures.

2.3 XML Formatting

One obstacle to mining full-text is the variation in the organization of articles used by different journals and publishers. A canonical representation has been generated, such that the majority of research articles can be represented by a six-section structure comprising *Title, Abstract, Introduction, Methods, Results, Discussion.* For example, *Materials and Methods, Experimental Procedures, Patients and Methods, Systems and Methods* are all tagged using the canonical form Methods. Figure 2 shows the XML structure following processing by GetItFull. The citation is similarly tagged by *Journal Name, Publication Year, Issue Number, Volume and Page Number.* This XML structure facilitates exporting the document to a database or other electronic information system for further processing and archiving. Once the various section tags are inserted, articles that do not conform to the six-section structure are identified. Such articles, for example editorials and letters to the editor, are stored separately and the user can choose whether or not to include them in a study.

```
<?xml version='1.0'?>
  <Doc>
    <Title>
      Title of the document here …
    </Title>
    <Abstract>
      Abstract of document here …
    </Abstract>
    <Introduction>
      Introduction of document here …
    </Introduction>
    <Methods>
      Materials and methods section of document here …
    </Methods>
    <Results>
      Results section of document here …
    </Results>
    <Discussion>
      Discussion section of document here …
    <Discussion>
  </Doc>
```

Fig. 2. The XML structure of a full-text article after GetItFull pre-processing

2.4 Article Pre-processing

Figures and images are not downloaded, and tables are converted to text, resulting in reduced download times and storage space. GetItFull performs a number of commonly used tasks needed for downloading and pre-processing of full-text documents including

- Connecting to the journal Web site;
- Downloading of HTML articles by reverse chronological order or by specified dates, and replacing of special symbols using standard-character coding (e.g. α with *alpha*);
- Removing of HTML tags and images;
- Conversion of tables into text;
- Deleting of references;
- Inserting article reference information, i.e., *Journal Name*, *Publication Year*, etc. as XML tags;
- Identification and extraction of article sections such as *Abstract*, *Introduction*, *Methods*, *Results*, *Discussion* and *figure legends/captions*;
- Removing of non-research articles such as *editorial, erratum, letters to editor*, etc.

2.5 Download Recovery

On exit GetItFull generates a configuration file that stores the address of the last issue downloaded. This allows the application to automatically resume the download on reconnection.

3 Applications and Limitations

GetItFull was developed as part of our current studies on the use of full-text mining for microarray gene annotation. The corpus for this study contained 20 journals (Table 1) from a 4-year period (2000-2003). Initially, PERL scripts were written to download and pre-process the articles. However, this proved to be extremely time-consuming and demonstrated the need for an integrated system.

Initial analysis of approximately 5 000 articles from two journals in the above list (Table 1) shows that abstracts contain only 34% of the information available from the full-text articles [18].

As a Windows-based application tool using the Internet Explore DOM interface, GetItFull runs only on the Microsoft Windows platform with Internet Explorer as its Web browser. In the current release, GetItFull will download all the articles from a site in a given time period. Whilst significantly faster than the PERL scripts, this is still a slow process, taking approximately two minutes to download and format each article (based on a Pentium processor with 512 MB RAM via a 2 MB Internet connection). Current developments include the incorporation of a query tool to provide the user with a more selective range of articles. Other developments include the incorporation of subscription journals, which would necessitate the user providing login details before accessing those journals. A further challenge to text mining in molecular biology and biomedicine is the identification of protein/gene names and their synonyms. The incorporation of a gene and protein synonym dictionary, which will replace these names with a unique identifier from Entrez-Gene [20], will improve the accuracy and sensitivity of subsequent mining procedures.

Table 1. List of downloaded journals and publisher's Web sites

Journal Name	URL
Biochemistry	http://pubs.acs.org/journals/bichaw/
BBRC	http://www.sciencedirect.com/science/journal/0006291X
Brain Research	http://www.sciencedirect.com/science/journal/00068993
Cancer	http://www3.interscience.wiley.com/cgi-in/jhome/28741
Cancer Research	http://cancerres.aacrjournals.org
Cell	http://www.cell.com/
EMBO Journal	http://embojournal.npgjournals.com/
FEBS Letters	http://www.sciencedirect.com/science/journal/00145793
Genes and Development	http://www.genesdev.org/
International Journal of Cancer	http://www3.interscience.wiley.com/cgi-in/jhome/29331
Journal of Biological Chemistry	http://www.jbc.org/
Journal of Cell Biology	http://www.jcb.org/
Journal of Neuroscience	http://www.jneurosci.org/
Nature	http://www.nature.com/
Neuron	http://www.neuron.org/
Neurology	http://www.neurology.org/
Nucleic Acid Research	http://nar.oupjournals.org/
Oncogene	http://www.nature.com/onc/
PNAS	http://www.pnas.org/
Science	http://www.sciencemag.org/

4   Discussion and Conclusions

The on-line provision of many high quality journals either through open access or via subscription means they have the potential to be automatically searched for information. However, the volume and complexity of the available literature also means that a keyword search is often not sufficiently specific, leading to the generation of too many results or missing important information. This has prompted many researchers to use text mining approaches to extract important and novel information from text. Knowledge discovery in text has therefore become an area of active research with new methods being continuously developed and assessed. Whilst initial text mining applications were based on abstracts, due in part to their ready availability, recent studies have demonstrated the advantages of using the full-text of documents [17,18]. The use of grid infrastructure to conduct text mining over distributed data and computational resources has also improved the efficiency of text-mining and thus the viability of mining larger and more complex documents such as full-text articles [21]. These developments have led to increased interest in mining full-text [22,23,24]. Whilst this research has demonstrated the value of using a corpus based on full-text articles, complete documents are more difficult to access, organize and analyze than abstracts. By pre-processing on-line journals, GetItFull provides the user with an XML document for each research article, facilitating the application of text-mining to full-text. The software and documentation is available from http://www.cthtech.com/products/gifpro/.

Acknowledgments

GetItFull is based on the software product GetItRight, a data migration tool from CTH Technologies. We are grateful to the GetItRight team and CTH technologies for allowing us to use their software.

References

1. Natarajan J., Berrar D., Hack C.J., and Dubitzky W.: Knowledge Discovery in Biology and Biotechnology Texts: A Review of Techniques, Evaluation Strategies, and Applications, Critical Reviews in Biotechnology, 25 (2005) 31-52
2. Hearst Marti, A.: Untangling text data mining, Proc. of ACL, 37 (1999)
3. Baeza-Yates, R., and Ribeiro-Nato, B.: Modern information retrieval, Addison-Wesley, Harlow, UK, (1999)
4. Ng, S-K., and Wong, M.: Towards routine automatic pathway discovery from on-line scientific text abstracts, Proceedings of the workshop on Genome Informatics, 10 (1999) 104-112
5. Wong, L.: A protein interaction extraction system, Pacific Symposium on Biocomputing, 6 (2001) 520-531
6. Park, J.C., Kim, H.S., and Kim, J.J.: Bi-directional incremental parsing for automatic pathway identification with combinatory categorical grammar, Pacific Symposium on Biocomputing 6 (2001) 396-407
7. Yakushiji, A., Tateisi, Y., Miyao, Y., and Tsujii, J.: Event extraction from biomedical papers using a full parser, Pacific Symposium on Biocomputing 6 (2001) 408-419
8. Friedman, C., Kra, P., Yu, H., Krauthammer, M., Rzhetsky, A.: GENIES: A natural language processing system for extraction of molecular pathways from journal article, Bioinformatics Suppl., 1 (2001) 74-82
9. Sekimizu, T., Park, H.S., and Tsujii, J.: Identifying the interaction between genes and gene products based on frequently seen verbs in MEDLINE abstracts, Proceedings of the workshop on Genome Informatics, (1998) 62-71
10. Rindflesch, T.C., Tanabe, L., Weinstein, J.N. and Hunter, L.: EDGAR: Extraction of drugs, genes, and relations from the biomedical literature. Pacific Symposium On Biocomputing, 5 (2000) 517-528
11. Craven, M., and Kumlien, J.: Constructing biological knowledge base by extracting information from text sources, Proceedings of the 7th International Conference on Intelligent Systems for Molecular Biology, (1999) 77-76
12. Stapley, B.J., Kelley, L.A., and Strenberg, M. J. E.: Predicting the sub-cellular location of proteins from text using support vector machines, Pacific Symposium on Biocomputing, 7 (2002) 374-385
13. Rindflesch, T.C., Rayan, J.V. and Hunter, L.: Extracting molecular binding relationships from biomedical text, Proc. App. Nat. Lan. Proc. and Ass. Comp. Ling., (2000) 188-195
14. Shah, P.K., Perz_Iratxeta, C., Bork P. and Andrade, M.A. Information Extraction from Full-text Scientific Articles, Where are the key words?, BMC Bioinformatics, 4 (20) (2003)
15. Yu, H., Hatzvisaailoulou, V., Friedman, C., Rzhetsky, A. and Wilbur, W. J. Automatic Extraction of Gene and Protein Synonyms from Medline and Journal Articles, Proceedings of AMIA Symposium, (2003) 919-23

16. Frideman, C., Kra, P., Yu, H., Krauthammer, M., and Rzhetsky, A.: Geneis: A Natural language processing system, Bioinformatics, 17 (2001) 74-82

17. Schuemie, M.J., Weeber, M., Schijvenaars, B.J.A., van Mulligen, E.M., van der Eijk, C.C., Jelier, R., Mons, B., and Kors, J.A. Distribution of Information in Biomedical Abstracts and Full-text Publications, Bioinformatics, 20 (2004) 2597-2604

18. Bremer, E.G., Natarajan, J. Zhang, Y., DeSesa, C., Hack, C.J. and Dubitzky, W. Text mining of full text articles and creation of a knowledge base for analysis of microarray data, Lecture Notes in Artificial Intelligence, Knowledge exploration in Life Science Informatics, (2004) 84-95

19. Microsoft Internet Transfer control help at http://support.microsoft.com/

20. Entrez-gene, a database of genes at http://www.ncbi.nih.gov/entrez/

21. Natarajan, J., Mulay, N., DeSesa, C., Hack, C.J., Dubitzky, W. and Bremer, E.G.: A Grid infrastructure for text mining of full text articles and creation of a knowledge base of gene relations, lecture Notes in Computer Science, Biological and Medical Data Analysis, 3745 (2005) 101 – 108

22. Text REtrieval Conference (TREC) home page at http://trec.nist.gov/

23. Cohen, K.B., Tanabe, L., Kinoshita, S. and Hunter, L.: A resource for constructing customized test suites for molecular biology entity identification system, Linking Biological Literature, Ontologies and Databases (Biolink 2004), (2004) 1-8

24. Müller, H.M., Kenny, E.E. and Sternberg, P.W.: Textpresso: An Ontology-Based Information Retrieval and Extraction System for Biological Literature, PLOS Biology, Vol. 2, Issue 11 (2004)

Author Index

Lecture Notes in Bioinformatics

Vol. 3886: E.G. Bremer, J. Hakenberg, E.-H.(S.) Han, D. Berrar, W. Dubitzky (Eds.), Knowledge Discovery in Life Science Literature. XIV, 147 pages. 2006.

Vol. 3745: J.L. Oliveira, V. Maojo, F. Martín-Sánchez, A.S. Pereira (Eds.), Biological and Medical Data Analysis. XII, 422 pages. 2005.

Vol. 3737: C. Priami, E. Merelli, P. Gonzalez, A. Omicini (Eds.), Transactions on Computational Systems Biology III. VII, 169 pages. 2005.

Vol. 3695: M.R. Berthold, R.C. Glen, K. Diederichs, O. Kohlbacher, I. Fischer (Eds.), Computational Life Sciences. XI, 277 pages. 2005.

Vol. 3692: R. Casadio, G. Myers (Eds.), Algorithms in Bioinformatics. X, 436 pages. 2005.

Vol. 3680: C. Priami, A. Zelikovsky (Eds.), Transactions on Computational Systems Biology II. IX, 153 pages. 2005.

Vol. 3678: A. McLysaght, D.H. Huson (Eds.), Comparative Genomics. VIII, 167 pages. 2005.

Vol. 3615: B. Ludäscher, L. Raschid (Eds.), Data Integration in the Life Sciences. XII, 344 pages. 2005.

Vol. 3594: J.C. Setubal, S. Verjovski-Almeida (Eds.), Advances in Bioinformatics and Computational Biology. XIV, 258 pages. 2005.

Vol. 3500: S. Miyano, J. Mesirov, S. Kasif, S. Istrail, P.A. Pevzner, M. Waterman (Eds.), Research in Computational Molecular Biology. XVII, 632 pages. 2005.

Vol. 3388: J. Lagergren (Ed.), Comparative Genomics. VII, 133 pages. 2005.

Vol. 3380: C. Priami (Ed.), Transactions on Computational Systems Biology I. IX, 111 pages. 2005.

Vol. 3370: A. Konagaya, K. Satou (Eds.), Grid Computing in Life Science. X, 188 pages. 2005.

Vol. 3318: E. Eskin, C. Workman (Eds.), Regulatory Genomics. VII, 115 pages. 2005.

Vol. 3240: I. Jonassen, J. Kim (Eds.), Algorithms in Bioinformatics. IX, 476 pages. 2004.

Vol. 3082: V. Danos, V. Schachter (Eds.), Computational Methods in Systems Biology. IX, 280 pages. 2005.

Vol. 2994: E. Rahm (Ed.), Data Integration in the Life Sciences. X, 221 pages. 2004.

Vol. 2983: S. Istrail, M.S. Waterman, A. Clark (Eds.), Computational Methods for SNPs and Haplotype Inference. IX, 153 pages. 2004.

Vol. 2812: G. Benson, R.D. M. Page (Eds.), Algorithms in Bioinformatics. X, 528 pages. 2003.

Vol. 2666: C. Guerra, S. Istrail (Eds.), Mathematical Methods for Protein Structure Analysis and Design. XI, 157 pages. 2003.